Walter Lübeck

L-Carnitine
"The Supernutrient for Fitness"

The Safe and Stress-Free Way to Manage Weight,
Increase Physical Performance and Mental Capacity, and
Build a Natural Immune-Protective Shield

Scientific Consultation:
Dr. Stefan Siebrecht, B.S. in Biochemistry

Translated by Christine M. Grimm

T0169282

LOTUS PRESS
SHANGRI-LA

Important Note: The information introduced in this book has been carefully researched and passed on to the best of our knowledge and conscience. Despite this fact, neither the author nor the publisher assume any type of liability for presumed or actual damages of any kind that might result from the direct or indirect application or use of the statements in this book. The information in this book is intended for educational purposes and is not to be understood as therapeutic or diagnostic instructions in the medical sense. Serious illnesses or any symptoms that may possibly conceal a serious ailment must absolutely be diagnosed and given therapeutical treatment by a healthcare practitioner. Since, particularly in the case of L-carnitine, the current state of knowledge expands almost every week through new studies, it is important to be informed about the latest status of the L-carnitine research and consult the most recent edition of this book.

The Author— Walter Lubeck Walter Lübeck has been active as a seminar leader for alternative methods of healing, holistic personality development, and success training since 1988. Since then, more than 8000 participants have attended his seminars, lectures, and workshops worldwide.

The results of Walter Lübeck's work have been made available to the broad public in his 19 books, which have been translated into 12 languages, and numerous articles in specialized magazines. His professional background includes training as a naturopath, 10 years of studying classical and complex homeopathy, as well as phytotherapy, NLP training, and more than 15 years of involvement with alternative therapies and healthy nutrition.

First English Edition 2000
©by Lotus Press
Box 325, Twin Lakes, WI 53181, USA
The Shangri-La Series is published in cooperation
with Schneelöwe Verlagsberatung, Federal Republic of Germany
©1998 by Windpferd Verlagsgesellschaft mbH, Aitrang, Germany
All rights reserved
Translated by Christine M. Grimm
Cover design by Kuhn Graphik, Digitales Design, Zürich
Interior pictures: on pages: 4, 5, 10, 21, 24, 26, 30, 32, 35, 38, 44, 47, 48, 58 by The Image Bank, Munich. Pictures on pages 15, 22 and 36 by Schneelöwe, Aitrang

ISBN 0-914955-59-4
Library of Congress Catalog Number 00-131344

Printed in Germany

Acknowledgments

The following have made a special contribution to the creation of this book:
Dr. Stefan Siebrecht and Hannes Pharma, Munich

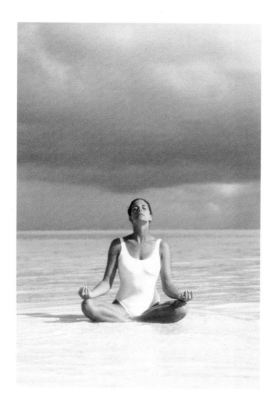

Table of Contents

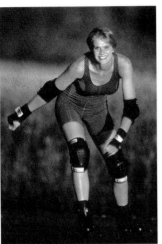

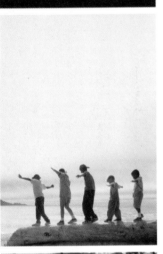

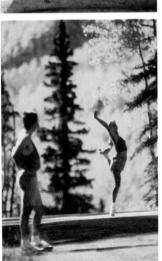

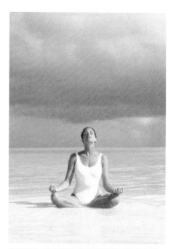

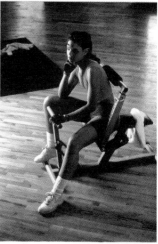

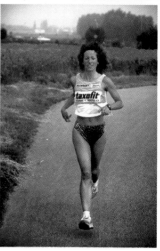

L-Carnitine Is Important for Everyone

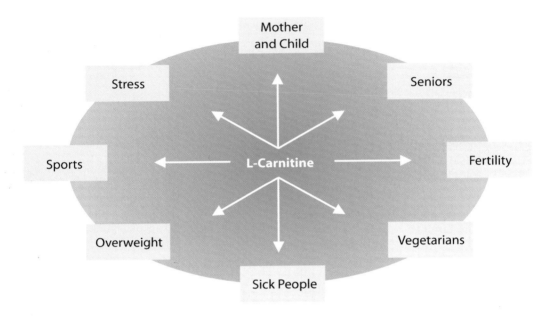

L-Carnitine

Muscles
- Increases strength and endurance
- Relieves physical and mental fatigue
- Promotes and maintains new development of muscle mass
- Reduces muscle injuries, sore muscles, stitches in the side
- Accelerates regeneration

Heart
- Increases cardiac output, force of the myocardial contraction, ATP production
- Lowers the heart rate under stress
- Reduces the intensity of cardiac infarction
- Reduces symptoms of heart failure, angina pectoris
- Increases heart exercise tolerance

Immune Cells
- Supplies energy to immune cells
- Increases activity of immune cells under stress
- Doesn't strain the immune system
- Positive effects, even during serious illnesses, for all those for whom other immune stimulants are contraindicated
- Can be used on long-term basis, no danger of overdose

Introduction

There is a natural substance that most people, with the exception of scientific specialists, (still) don't know about. Many experts say that it is currently the best-researched dietary supplement in the world and has every appearance of—almost—being a wonder remedy. Moreover, it is non-toxic, without contraindications and adverse interactions, and well-tolerated by both young and old.

It's hard to believe.

But true!

This substance is called *L-carnitine* and has been a personal tip among top athletes for years. It helps the body achieve a holistically oriented increase of its performance potential and clearly stabilizes the psyche, even during all types of extreme strain. The unpleasant accompanying effects of intensive physical training, such as sore muscles and subsequent phases of physical and mental exhaustion, are reduced. Susceptibility to injury during top athletic performances may also decrease.

I first encountered L-carnitine when the friendly trainer at "my" fitness club asked me if I wanted to try drinking "something different" for once. They were having a special offer on L-carnitine drinks. "What kind of stuff is that?" I asked. "Really sounds like it's something chemical. Is it good for me?" I couldn't resist feeling somewhat mistrustful at the sound of the name. "No problem!" she said with a smile. "L-carnitine is natural and makes people really fit in a healthy way. In addition, it can effectively help you lose weight—if you train on a regular basis. And you'll build up better musculature. And you can pretty much forget sore muscles and exhaustion after training. Give it a try. I just learned all about it at an advanced training seminar and checked it out for myself. It really makes sense to take it!"

I couldn't say "no" to so much friendly competence and took her advice. Moreover, she had already helped me with her expertise on more than one occasion. In terms of training theory and sport nutrition, Sonja couldn't be fooled that easily. She also recommended that I additionally use the L-carnitine lozenges.

"Okay," I thought to myself later as I drank a glass of "L-Carnitine & Minerals." It doesn't taste different than anything else. I can't find any objections to it. The surprises then

L-carnitine—almost a wonder remedy?

Also read the interview with the overall world-record holder in the Quintuple Ironman Triathlon, Astrid Benohr, in the Appendix I, on page 67.

L-carnitine increases the body's performance potential and stabilizes the psyche.

came when I worked out afterward. My favorite exercises of the stationary bike and Stairmaster were definitely less exerting—and I was better at them! Even while working on the weight machines, I noticed clear improvements. And the next day, despite a three-week break because of vacation, I hardly had any sore muscles after the intensive training. Curious, I began to research what this stuff with the funny name was all about. What I discovered about it was—and still is—fascinating.

Immediately noticeable results.

Because I believe that this substance shouldn't just be reserved for top athletes and managers, I have compiled what I think are the truly significant facts on L-carnitine for the user.

Read it and you will probably be astonished.

And then try L-carnitine yourself. This is what convinces most people since L-carnitine noticeably increases their level of fitness within a short amount of time. If you don't want to neglect the quality of your life, despite all the demands of our era, you will find this modern nutritive supplement to be a valuable aid.

Convince yourself of the positive effects!

In addition, there are an entire series of scientific studies clearly proving that L-carnitine supports health and healing in a multitude of health disorders.

I hope you enjoy some entertaining and informative hours with this book.

Walter Tusbed

L-Carnitine—The Energy Supplier

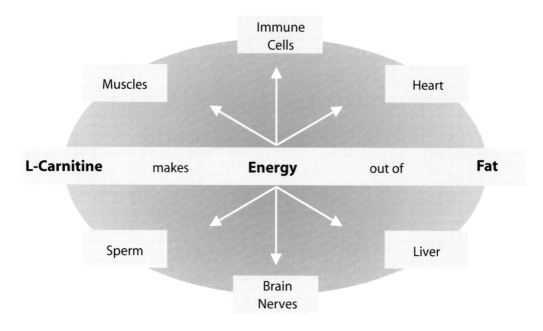

L-Carnitine

Brain Nerves	• Slows aging of brain, dementia, Alzheimer's disease • Improves cognitive abilities like concentration, memory, and ability to learn • Reduces loss of receptors • Accelerates renewal of tissue
Liver	• Improves liver function • Increases protein synthesis and the liver's fat-burning process • Reduces problems of fatty liver • Accelerates renewal of liver tissue
Sperm	• Improves activity of sperm • Enlarges amount and number of sperm • Increases fertility of sperm

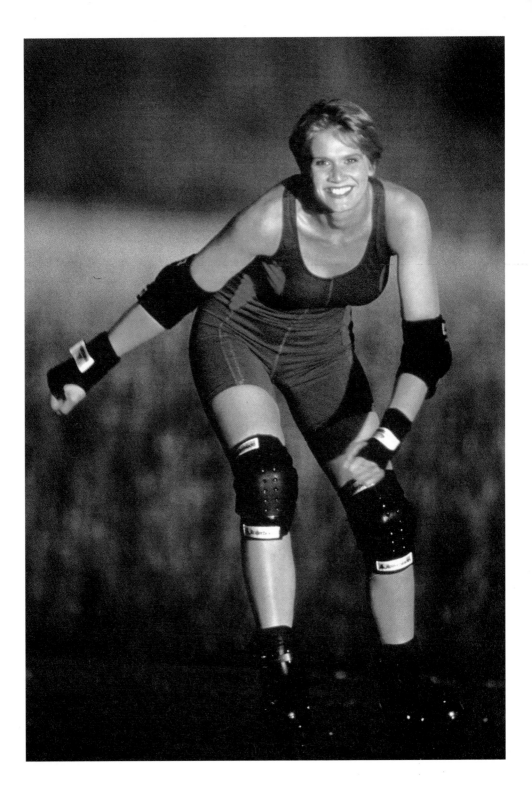

Chapter 1

What Is L-Carnitine?

L-carnitine was discovered at the beginning of the 20th century by the Russian scientists Gulewitsch and Krimberg. However, a long period of time passed before its commercial use as an affordable dietary supplement began. The main reason for the decades of delay was the high cost of producing the minor amount of this substance that was available from meat. On the other hand, a constantly increasing number of interesting research reports listed the many versatile applications of L-carnitine as an outstandingly well-tolerated vitamin-like dietary supplement with the structure rather similar to that of an amino acid. It only became possible to make L-carnitine available to everyone in large amounts at moderate prices during the 1980s, when completely new processes *not* based on the raw material of meat went into production. At about the same time, there was a drastic increase in the number of scientific papers on the functions of L-carnitine in metabolism. This research revealed its possible applications for maintaining normal life functions, supporting the healing of various health disorders, and improving quality of life. In 1998, there were already more than 9000(!) academic research reports on L-carnitine. About 300 more are published throughout the world every year. The limits of how this dietary supplement can be used for the benefit of humanity are still far from being fully explored.

L-carnitine first became available to the public at moderate prices during the 1980s.

Also for the benefit of animals! Many pets, like cats and dogs, are treated with L-carnitine as a well-tolerated accompanying remedy against many diseases and to maintain or improve vitality.

The Following Basic Statements Can Be Made about L-Carnitine Today:

➤ It is an essential component of nutrition for more highly developed animal organisms.
➤ It is a completely natural substance that can mainly be found in the (muscle) flesh. Eggs and milk (products) contain little of it. Fruit contains minor amounts, and very little of this substance is generally found in vegetables and nuts.
➤ Since it is a vitamin-like nutrient related to the vitamins of the B group in terms of its effects, L-carnitine was also called vitamin B_T for a time. Scientists still disagree about the

Animal Products/ Average Values		Plant Products/Average Values	
	mg/kg		mg/kg
Crab	9000	Applesauce	31
Sheep	2100	Tomatoes	29
Goat	1700	Pears	27
Lamb	780	Brewer's yeast	24
Beef	700	Rice	18
Sheep's heart	500	Peaches	16
Pork	300	Asparagus	13
Rabbit	210	Avocados	13
Beef heart	200	Peas	12
Ewe's milk	140	Grapefruit	11
Rabbit liver	100	Wheat germ	10
Poultry	80	Bread, green beans	8
Pork liver	50	Cauliflower, Peanuts	1
Beef liver	25	Potatoes, oranges	0
Cow's milk	25	Spinach, carrots	0
Beef kidney	20	Cabbage	0
Chicken egg	8		

Occurrence of L-carnitine in food

L-carnitine— vitamin or not?

definition of vitamins. Originally, vitamins were defined as those nutrients that the body couldn't produce itself. However, as the respective state of knowledge has improved through the years, it has become apparent that various vitamins are produced in certain amounts by metabolism itself. Consequently, many experts now tend to perceive vitamins to be substances that are absolutely necessary for maintaining life functions—no matter where they come from. In this respect, L-carnitine can definitely be called the "forgotten" vitamin of the B group.

➤ According to the international classification by nutritional scientists, L-Carnitine is listed right after choline, another vitamin-like substance.

➤ It is a substance that is absolutely required for normal life processes of the organism. It is necessary for the body's own (endogenous) energy production and for normal fat metabolism. This is why it can be found in practically every area of the organism. It occurs in larger amounts wherever an abundance of energy is necessary for maintaining normal bodily functions.

There is only a total of four substances that are considered to be "vitamin-like" and listed in the "Handbook of Vitamins," the bible for experts on vital substances. These are: choline, taurine, inositol, and L-carnitine. Note: choline is now classed as an essential nutrient in the USA.

➤ L-carnitine can be produced in the human liver, the kidneys, and the brain. However, only about ten percent of the normal requirement can be covered with this amount!

Organ	mg/kg	µmol/ml;g
Skeletal muscles	19,000	3.96
Liver	650	2.90
Heart	220	4.80
Kidneys	60	1.00
Brain	80	0.30
Plasma	30	0.05
Erythrocytes		0.24
Lymphocytes		1.00
Epididymis		60-65
Ejaculate		0.3-5.0

Occurrence of L-carnitine in the human body

The substantial remaining portion must be absorbed through food from the outside. Infants produce no L-carnitine in their own metabolism. With increasing age, the ability to produce L-carnitine slowly develops. This is why children, in order to grow up healthy, are much more dependent upon the carnitine in food than adults. Only after the age of about 15 years does the endogenous (body's own) L-carnitine synthesis function to the full extent in the human body. Appropriate attention must definitely be paid to this factor if children are raised as vegetarians. For this, as well as other important reasons, I urgently advise you to at least give them adequate amounts of eggs and milk (products) or L-carnitine as a nutrtional supplement if they don't have any meat in their diets. Otherwise, developmental and growth disorders like anemia, learning difficulties, and dysfunctions of the immune system may occur. Under these circumstances, lasting damage cannot be ruled out.

➤ L-carnitine makes a substantial and greatly varied contribution, both directly and indirectly, to normal functioning of the overall metabolism. It can improve vitality (energy metabolism), it helps prevent heart problems and help heal them, and slow down the aging process in some respects. It therefore makes an important contribution to a high quality of life in the mature years, strengthen the male reproductive capability, and offers substantial support to the immune system, the formation of blood, and the deoxygenation of the red blood cells. It helps prevent strokes and relieve their consequences, as well as promoting detoxification. It also helps protect the cells against many harmful substances and the formation of tumors.

The body contains about 25,000 milligrams—however, metabolism can only produce about 16 milligrams per day.

Children need L-carnitine from their food in order to grow up healthy.

L-carnitine improves metabolic function.

A Summary of the History of L-Carnitine

1905

L-carnitine was discovered by the Russian researchers *Gulewitsch* and *Krimberg* in meat extract from the muscular meat of mammals. They discovered that this substance is absolutely necessary for the biochemical functioning of the muscle cells. The name is derived from the Latin *carnis* (meat).

1927

The chemical structure of L-carnitine, which the scientist Krimberg had already theoretically determined at the time of discovery, was confirmed by experimentation.

1935

The scientist *Strack* researched the functions of L-carnitine in comparison to *choline*, which is related in terms of its chemical structure.

1947

The scientist *Fraenkel* carried out research in terms of the undiscovered vitamins of the B group. Most of the vitamins of the B group (thiamin, riboflavin, niacin, pyridoxine, pantothenic acid, biotin, and folic acid) were discovered by 1946. L-carnitine also played a role in this project.

Mealworms are very well suited for studies on vitamins and vitamin-like substances since, in a certain sense, their organism behaves in a manner similar to that of human beings.

1952

In his research regarding substances necessary for life in the nutrition of mealworms, Fraenkel discovered that L-carnitine is a component of the nutrition necessary for their lives. Within this context, he isolated L-carnitine from human liver and gave it the name "Vitamin B_T." Even today, many specialists view L-carnitine as a "forgotten" vitamin of the B group.

1958

The researcher *Fritz* discovered that L-carnitine may increase the burning of fatty acids in the mitochondria of cells. In the scientific world, this perception established L-carnitine as a fundamental factor in the burning of fat in human metabolism.

At the beginning of the 1980s
Revolutionary new processes were developed for mass-production of this supplement. As a result, L-carnitine became available in an even quality, completely independent of "meat" as its raw material. In this form, it is easy to store and use in a variety of ways. In addition, it became much more affordable. Consequently, it is now available to all health-oriented people as a dietary supplement.

1980
At the Olympics, the Italian endurance athletes celebrated their first big success, which can mostly be attributed to the use of L-carnitine. The Italian Olympic team was the only one to take L-carnitine as a dietary supplement at that time.

1982
At the World Soccer Championship, Italy's team became the unsurpassed world champion. In this competition as well, the Italian team was the only one to use L-carnitine.

1986
Instead of the previous chemical process, a production method that is biotechnological and close to the workings of nature was developed by the Swiss company LONZA. This production method does not employ gene manipulation.

1980 to today
Throughout the world, extensive studies are being carried out on the functions of L-carnitine in the metabolism of human beings and animals. Its possible application as a bioactive dietary supplement and accompanying therapeutic agent in a multitude of health disorders is also being researched.
Among other problems, this includes: Alzheimer's disease, AIDS, heart attack, stroke, muscle disorders, diabetes, sepsis (blood poisoning), post-polio syndrome, and cirrhosis of the liver.

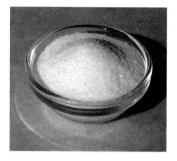

In terms of its appearance, L-carnitine looks like powdered sugar.

There is no legal limit assigned in the USA regarding the daily dosages of additional L-carnitine. However, it has been proven that dosages of three to six grams per day are completely safe and beneficial for the metabolism in times when greater demands are placed on the body.

➤ The human body contains about 20 to 25 grams of L-carnitine.

➤ The normal daily requirement of L-carnitine is between 200 mg and 500 mg. When subject to intense physical strain or stress, the daily requirement for L-carnitine may easily increase to 1,200 milligrams. Top athletes supplement with up to nine grams of the substance per day to stabilize their ability to perform and reduce their risk of injury during competition.

➤ Only about ten percent of the daily amount of L-carnitine required can be supplied by the body's own production. However, about 30 grams of protein are needed to produce just one gram of L-carnitine. This means that protein metabolism may also be quickly overstrained when the diet includes too little L-carnitine and protein. This applies particularly when there is a high level of physical demands. If a much greater amount of L-carnitine is required in stressful situations, additional amounts of this vital substance must be supplied through the diet or as a dietary supplement since the body cannot further increase its own production of L-carnitine.

Only about ten percent of the daily requirement can be covered by the endogenous (body's own) L-carnitine synthesis.

L-Carnitine

D-Carnitine

D-carnitine is injurious to health.

L-Carnitine and D-Carnitine

Carnitine exists in two chemical formulas that are the same, D-carnitine and L-carnitine. The only difference is that D-carnitine is structured as the mirror image of L-carnitine. The consequence of this small but significant difference is that D-carnitine has a toxic effect in relation to various bodily functions. In addition, it proves to have almost none of the health-promoting qualities of its sister substance L-carnitine. Before the new production process for carnitine was developed at the beginning of the 1980s, the so-called D/L-carnitine was on the market for a time. This substance is a mixture of both types of carnitine, which is quite inexpensive to manufacture. After the health-impairing characteristics of D-carnitine were discovered, the U.S. FDA banned the sale of this substance as a dietary supplement. Today, the carnitine offered for commercial sale is *always* L-carnitine. Note: The human organism only produces L-carnitine.

Symptoms of an L-Carnitine Deficiency

• *Deposits of fat droplets (triglycerides) in the tissue*
• *Fatty degeneration of tissue in heart, liver, muscles (lipidosis)*
• *Rapid exhaustion and decrease in vitality*
• *Muscle weakness, muscle atrophy, fatigue*
• *Longer recovery periods after strain*
• *Weakening of immune system*
• *Deterioration of blood parameters (Hct, Hb values)*
• *Decreased activity of male sperm cells and infertility*
• *Growth disorders in children*
• *Heart disease, heart failure, dysrhythmia, angina pectoris*
• *Fatty degeneration of liver, cirrhosis of the liver, liver-function disturbances*
• *Reduction of protein synthesis*
• *Increased susceptibility toward metabolic toxins such as ammonia and various environmental toxins, as well as free radicals*

Hct = hematocrit (number of red blood cells);
Hb = hemoglobin (the oxygen carrying molecule in red blood cells, that delivers oxygen to all the cells that need it).

➤ Health problems, stress, pregnancy, breastfeeding, and intense physical strain can dramatically increase the need for L-carnitine.

➤ The symptoms of an L-carnitine deficiency are diverse and non-specific. A lack of this vitamin-like substance can basically only be determined through a carefully directed, quite complicated diagnosis procedure. For example, there is usually no relationship between the L-carnitine level in the blood serum and that of the cells. In other words: If the blood is examined for an L-carnitine deficiency and the values are normal, there may still be a deficiency of L-carnitine in the cells—with the corresponding disharmonious effects on health and vitality. For certain heart diseases, increased levels of L-carnitine values in the blood serum are even typical!

How Does L-Carnitine Work?

Summarized in three points, it can be said of L-carnitine's main field of action that

- It gives the body strength in an extensive manner
- It supports the ability to deal with (high-level) physical and psychological performance, in both the short- and long-term(!), in a way that avoids wear tear, and is especially effective physiologically.
- It protects the mind and nervous system, as well as promoting their functions

L-carnitine mainly increases the rate at which fat is "burned".

Wherever the organism needs energy, it plays an important role. For example, it transports fatty acids into the mitochondria, the biochemical powerhouses in the interior of the cells. However, L-carnitine not only participates in fat metabolism. Even when energy is acquired from proteins or carbohydrates, it contributes to the respective reactions. However, when there are adequate amounts of it, it primarily is involved in producing energy from fat.

In every respect, this fuel is much more effective for the organism than both of the other alternatives. When they are burned, fats deliver about six times as much energy as glucose or proteins. Moreover, when energy is stored in the form of glucose, the same proportions of weight in water are necessary to store the glucose in the body as a quickly available fuel reserve. When protein is burned, for example, the extremely harmful metabolic toxin *ammonia* is created, among other things.

Only by burning fat can energy effectively be made available to a larger extent and for a longer period of time.

Furthermore, L-carnitine promotes the functioning of the immune system by giving the macrophages (the large phagocytic cells) the strength to move quickly through the body when they hunt after unwelcome intruders like viruses, bacteria, or fungi. As guardians of the metabolism, their ability to coat troublemakers and literally eat them up is also effectively supported by L-carnitine.

The male sperm cells must have a great deal of mobility and endurance to reach an egg cell (ovum) and be capable of fertilizing it. The required energy for this process is also provided by an adequate supply of L-carnitine. In a certain sense, L-carnitine could be called a male fertility agent.

The Body Can Produce Minor Amounts of L-Carnitine on Its Own

Human metabolism has the ability to produce L-carnitine on its own from various starting materials. The main "factory" for this task is in the body's unbelievably versatile chemical laboratory, the liver. Further minor amounts are synthesized in the kidneys and the brain. In order for the manufacturing process to work at all, certain substances are absolutely necessary as the starting materials.

These are: vitamin C, vitamin B_3 (niacin), vitamin B_6, B_{12}, folic acid, iron, and the essential amino acids lysine and methionine. In addition, five different enzymes are required for the synthesis of L-carnitine. If a deficiency of just *one* of these substances occurs, the body's own synthesis of L-carnitine is reduced.

Furthermore, a lack of vitamin C is the first thing to lead to symptoms of L-carnitine deficiency because the endogenous production of L-carnitine no longer functions in this case.

Endogenous L-carnitine production is only completely capable of functioning when a person is about 15 years old. It is practically non-existent in small children. Even the bodies of adults can only produce about ten percent of the normal daily requirement of L-carnitine from metabolism itself. This is why an additional supply through the diet is very important. This applies particularly when there are above-average physical or psychological strains to deal with or other circumstances, such as illness, that lead to an increased need for L-carnitine.

Amino acids are the simplest building blocks of proteins. They are the basis from which a larger protein of the body tissue, such as the musculature, is built. As substances necessary for life, "essential amino acids" are those that must be supplied through the diet since the body is not capable of producing them on its own.

Also see the information under the question "Who Particularly Needs This Dietary Supplement?" on page 63.

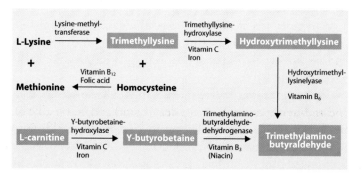

Biosynthesis of L-carnitine (I).

> ## Biosynthesis of L-Carnitine (II)
>
> - *Low capacity (approx. 16-20 mg/d = 100 μmol = 1.2 μmol/d/ kg of body weight)*
> - *Only about 10% of daily requirement comes from the endogenous synthesis*
> - *No adaptation or increase occurs when the body has an additional need for L-carnitine*
> - *Synthesis is dependent upon vitamin A, B_3, B_6, B_{12}, C iron, folic acid, lysine, and methionine, as well as five enzymes.*
> - *Lack of these components restricts the synthesis*
> - *The five steps of synthesis only possible in the liver when there are adequate amounts of the necessary components*
> - *Full activity of synthesis is only possible when 15 year of age has been reached*
> - *The synthesis output diminishes with age*
> - *Many people do not have an L-carnitine synthesis that meets their daily requirement*
> - *L-carnitine supplementation has no harmful influence on the body's own synthesis*

A large reserve of L-carnitine increases vitality, as well as the ability to deal with all kinds of stress in a well-balanced way. This is an important help in healing the LSD syndrome, which in recent decades has spread increasingly among the people in Western industrial nations. No—the topic isn't drugs here. In this case, the abbreviation "LSD" doesn't mean lysergic acid diethylamide, but *low sexual desire*. As science has discovered, the many stressful environmental influences and everyday strains sometimes strongly subdue many people's lustful desires. This not only means a substantial reduction in the quality of life, but also brings with it many kinds of long-term damage to social life and health.

As a healthy remedy for staying fit, L-carnitine can make a contribution by strengthening the ability of coping with strain and improving the capacity for dealing with stress in a balanced manner.

Its strengthening effect applies for more than just the mind: L-carnitine detoxifies the cells and the mitochondria. These biochemical powerhouses in the interior of the cell can also transform many different substances into others and thereby keep metabolism running. L-carnitine not only protects the

Endotoxins, such as ammonia, are toxins created by metabolism in the body. Necroses are cells that have died.

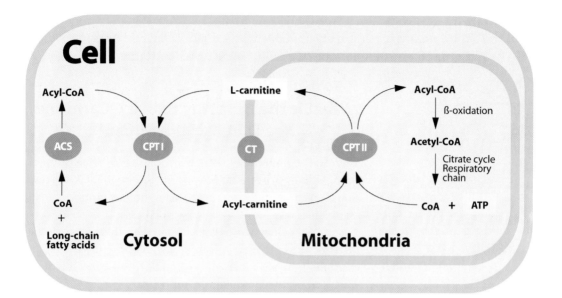

Cell

Acyl-CoA →   L-carnitine ←   Acyl-CoA

↑   ↓ ß-oxidation

(ACS)   (CPT I)   (CT)   (CPT II)   Acetyl-CoA

↑   Citrate cycle / Respiratory chain ↓

CoA ←   Acyl-carnitine →   CoA + ATP
+
Long-chain fatty acids   **Cytosol**   **Mitochondria**

---

cell membranes against damage through acids, endotoxins, tumors, necrosis, and stress factors, as well as free radicals, and optimizes them in their metabolic functions—it also promotes the repair of damaged cell membranes. L-carnitine most intensively helps the immune cells, the erythrocytes (red blood cells) and the sperm (sperm cells).

A further important effect is protecting the nervous system against the metabolic poison *ammonia*. Not only is this produced during intensive physical strain as a waste product of fat metabolism, but also in functional disorders of the liver: for example, in relation to chronic abuse of alcohol or when hepatitis occurs in larger concentrations. L-carnitine continues to support the healing of damaged nerve cells.

For red blood cells, L-carnitine is absolutely necessary for life. It detoxifies them from the end products of metabolism, which cannot be made harmless in any other manner. At the same time, it increases their life span, improves their ability to supply the cells with oxygen, and makes sure that they don't stick to each other as easily. This helps avoid thrombosis, strokes, and heart attacks. It improves the overall fluidity of the blood and therefore its ability to reach all possible areas of the body through the fine blood capillaries. This supports the blood's function of delivering nutrients and picking up the end products of metabolism so they can be disposed of. This process is the only way a healthy organism can be maintained.

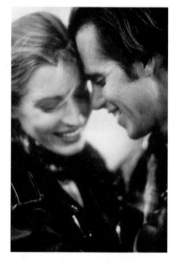

L-carnitine strengthens the immune system and provides energy for the male sperm cells.

Some readers may think that all the positive functions attributed to L-carnitine are exaggerated. But these are the facts. All of this, and even more, has been scientifically proven for years.

What Is the Best Way to Use L-Carnitine as a Dietary Supplement?

In situations of intense strain, such as those that top athletes must deal with, considerably higher individual doses can be used. However, individual doses of more than 5 grams are pointless.

With all the good things that L-carnitine has to offer, the question naturally arises as to how it can best be used as a dietary supplement. Simply acting according to the motto of "a lot helps a lot" is especially pointless in the case of L-carnitine.

You can achieve an optimal absorbtion through the small intestine into the metabolism by dividing the daily dose, for example, into several small portions. Knowledgeable nutritional experts recommend an individual dose of something like 100 to 500 milligrams, for example. However, L-carnitine should not be taken together with the protein drinks that are so popular in fitness sports. The simultaneous presence of

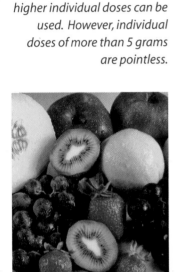

For the best absorption into the organism, take it with fruit or vegetables.

Absorption of L-Carnitine in the Tissue
• The cells contain 100 ml more L-carnitine than the blood
➤ An active transport into the cells is necessary
➤ 80% of the L-carnitine in the heart is actually resorbed
➤ Satiable, energy-dependent, sodium-dependent
➤ Lack of energy in the cells leads to a reduced absorption of L-carnitine and a decrease of the L-carnitine concentration in the cells; for example, in the heart-muscle cells during heart failure
➤ Passive absorption is possible at higher concentrations
• Long-term oral supplementation increases the L-carnitine content of all tissues, cells, and body fluids.

larger amounts of amino acids can hinder the absorption of L-carnitine in your digestive tract!

If you want to take L-carnitine so that its full effect is available at a certain point in time, such as your training period or an important competition, do so about two hours beforehand. The main effective period is between two and six hours after it has been taken, as discovered in experiments with athletes. However, L-carnitine shouldn't be taken after 4 p.m. Other-

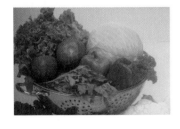

wise, it could interfere with the nightly rest phases by keeping you awake at the wrong time and increasing your urge for activity! On the other hand, taking L-carnitine in the morning, right after you get up, or before lunch will increase your mental and physical alertness and vitality at exactly the right time.

Absorption of L-Carnitine over 24-Hour Period

	Time	30 mg/kg	100 mg/kg
• *Table according to Rizza (1993)*			
• *Values given in μmol/litre*			
(30 mg/kg 2g at 70 kg,	*0*	*0.00*	*0.00*
10 mg (kg 7 g L-carnitine)	*0.5*	*5.11*	*5.40*
• *1 g L-carnitine per day over*	*1*	*6.20*	*14.92*
120 days leads to a	**2**	**23.69**	**65.05**
stabilization of the carnitine	**3**	**27.10**	**90.74**
pool in athletes (Arenas 1991)	**4**	**25.72**	**88.32**
• *2 g L-carnitine per day leads to*	*5*	*23.00*	*72.32*
an increase of the total	*6*	*18.50*	*50.43*
carnitine and free carnitine	*8*	*9.30*	*35.79*
in muscles after 28 days	*10*	*7.20*	*32.21*
(Neary 1992)	*12*	*4.50*	*17.43*
	14	*4.00*	*15.37*
• **Highest values 2-4 hours**	*18*	*2.60*	*9.69*
after taking L-carnitine	*24*	*0.20*	*4.09*

Summary

- *L-carnitine is a natural, vitamin-like and aminoacid-like substance*
- *L-carnitine is not a drug but a healthy dietary supplement*
- *L-carnitine has no harmful side effects and poses no known risks*
- *L-carnitine promotes and supports health in all phases of life*
- *L-carnitine deficiency is widespread but diagnosed only in extreme cases.*
- *Many people suffer from an L-carnitine deficiency without knowing it and sometimes they might not recognize the deficiency symptoms*
- *L-carnitine has positive effects on many health disorders*

➤ ***Many people could benefit from L-carnitine**

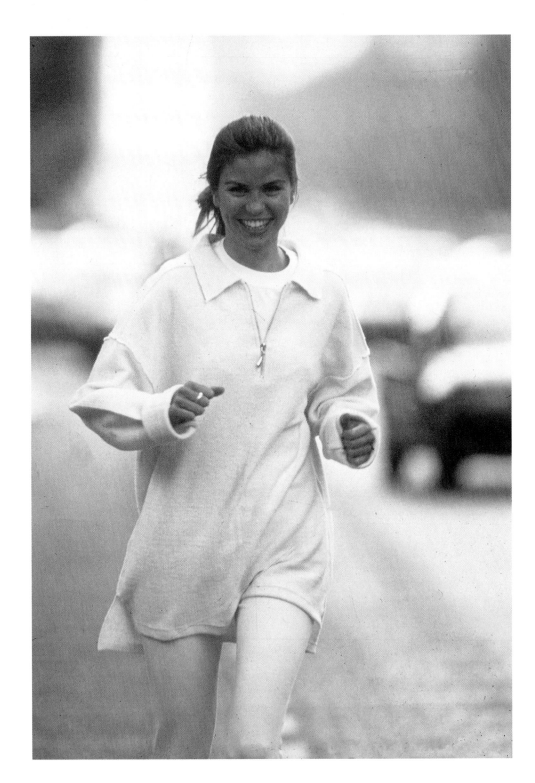

Chapter 2

The Healthy and Stress-Free Way to Manage Weight

Some people have no problems with their figure. Somehow, they are just naturally slender and would have a hard time gaining weight—others don't really worry about how they look, for one reason or another. And then there are people like me and perhaps even you.

It's not that there aren't enough diets and well-meant bits of advice, which often come from people who tend not to need any kind of slimming treatment anyway. Even weight-loss clinics and enormous amounts of teas, drops, pills, powders, and plasters could help. Theoretically, at least. I'm familiar with some of the fast weight-loss methods. I'm even thoroughly acquainted with most of the treatments that are naturally slow and therefore more lasting. After years of trying different approaches, I have developed a method for myself that is practicl and beneficial for my individual health and keeps my constitutional tendency toward excess pounds in check. In addition to a delicious whole-food diet, a fitness program that fits into my everyday life and is therefore easy to do on a regular basis, as well as a constructive attitude toward life, this method includes special nutritional supplements. Being slender is strongly related to emotional equilibrium—but it is equally dependent upon a harmoniously functioning metabolism. For example, anyone who is too weary (not lazy!) to participate in sports and experiences fitness exercises as torment, urgently needs support for his or her body. Otherwise, not even a very well-balanced emotional state will help.

An entire series of my books deals with how to develop and strengthen the psyche in its capacities. (These titles are listed in the *Bibliography*, on page 74.)

Here I would like to go into more detail about how the latest findings of L-carnitine research can be used within the scope of common weight-normalization practices to increase your vitality and help you become slender—and stay that way.

Yes—honestly—it does exist: the turbo-slim plaster. But it doesn't work! Except perhaps in terms of slimming down your wallet. But who wants to lose weight there!

Fasting

Increase vitality, become slim—and stay slim!

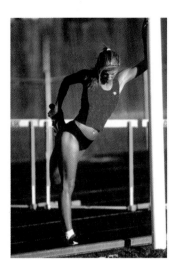

Fasting is often easier with like-minded people and supportive activities.

A fast that is carried out properly has always been an excellent means of purifying the body and losing weight. However, it is important to have the fast accompanied by an experienced physician, healing practitioner, or qualified nutritional specialist. Some people have physical ailments that must be taken into consideration when designing an individual fasting treatment so that no new health problems result. Often, it is easier to fast with a group of like-minded people. An optimal approach is to accompany the fast with some kind of self-awareness exercises, artistic activities, gymnastics, Tai Chi, Qi Gong, Yoga, or Reiki, for example.

Intestinal cleansing, plenty of fluids, adequate rest, and massages that promote detoxification are important aids in fasting. If the treatment takes place during vacation, the frequently occurring tiredness and exhaustion are certainly bothersome but not really tragic. However, the situation is different if you fast parallel to your everyday working life, filled with its many tasks and stressful moments: You can hardly afford constant tiredness and an inability to deal with things on the mental and physical level. In part, we can compensate for unpleasant accompanying symptoms by taking suitable vitamin/mineral preparations and doing the activities mentioned above. L-carnitine can also make a further important contribution here since it plays a key role in supplying energy with in the metabolism. When fasting, the decreasing amount of energy available from day to day because of the reduced food supply (even though the body attempts to eliminate as little of its precious substances as possible by increasing the rate of absorption in the kidneys) results in an inevitable reduction of the L-carnitine level. This adds to a general state of weakness. The euphoria that frequently occurs during such a fast should not be confused with an actual increase in capabilities.

Supplying L-carnitine as a dietary supplement supports vitality and makes it possible for someone to enjoy fasting while carrying on the normal daily activities since the remaining demands can be fulfilled as well. Specialists recommend at least 1,000 mg daily, depending on your body weight and level of external strain. Due to physiological reasons, lower daily doses do not achieve satisfactory results. By experimenting a bit, you can quickly discover the individual dosage most suitable for you.

The best approach is to divide the daily amount into three or four portions taken between right after you get up and early afternoon. Then the "fitness effect" of L-carnitine is immediately available when the highest degree of vital energy is required on the one hand. On the other hand, the increased supply of energy resulting from L-carnitine, which is often accompanied by a certain eagerness for work, won't disturb the nightly sleep. To discover the optimal timing for the L-carnitine effect, please remember: The "window" of the maximum effect lies between two and six hours after taking the supplement.

Because of its key role in supplying energy to the body, L-carnitine plays an important role in fasting.

The timing is important for the optimal effect.

Fasting Dissolves Fat Pads

In relation to fasting, a further important effect of taking additional L-carnitine is that fat metabolism is optimized. Without an adequate supply of L-carnitine, after a few days the body will fall back on energy production from the burning of proteins. However, the metabolic toxin ammonia is automatically produced as well in the process. The resulting additional strain on the organism leads to feelings of listlessness, the nerves are no longer as strong, and the liver has an additional burden placed on it. L-carnitine puts the body in the position of burning the existing fat deposits more intensely—one of the main effects that people want when they fast. This helps to dissolve the fat pads and eliminated together with the toxins and waste materials stored in the fat cells. Be sure to drink enough fluids when you fast—at best in the form of water. Approximate value: about 1 ounce of water per every kilo (2.2 pounds) of body weight every day. (Example: 150 pounds = 68 kilos = 68 ounces = approx. 2 quarts.) Don't try to fast "dry"!

L-carnitine can help to protect the cells and organs from being damaged by the harmful substances that are released. At the same time, the musculature is maintained because it doesn't have to serve as the "emergency fuel" and research indicates that up to ten percent more fat is burned. Furthermore, the versatile L-carnitine buffers the sensitive nervous system against the toxic ammonia: Since it has a certain chemical similarity with the harmful substance, but happens to be completely harmless, L-carnitine attaches itself to the same nerve connections that would otherwise be the target for the destructive effects of ammonia. Now that a friendly guest occupies the nerve cells, the toxic ammonia can no longer do harm to them.

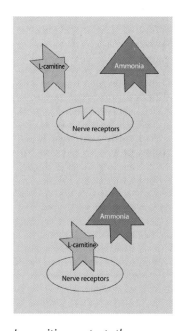

L-carnitine protects the nerve receptors against the neurotoxin ammonia. Ammonia blocks and lames the nerves, causing fatigue. In extreme cases like cirrhosis or cancer of the liver, it can cause coma and death through hepatic encephalopathy (brain failure caused by the loss of important liver functions).

Weight-Management Diet

Fasting isn't always the solution for weight problems. Today, nutritional science has developed a series of tailor-made diets to make managing weight easier. However, no matter how well the diet is put together, there can still easily be an L-carnitine deficiency. This applies particularly in stress and strain situations. With a diet, there is less to eat and the meat dishes that contain L-carnitine are included much less frequently or not at all because of their high number of calories. In addition, meat isn't necessarily the right food for a purification treatment. Doing without it for a while is sensible in helping the body clean house.

L-carnitine helps in burning the fat deposits—and protects the body against the harmful substances that are released.

Effects on Metabolism

- *L-carnitine is essential for the transport of long-chain fatty acids into the mitochondria. Without L-carnitine, long-chain fatty acids can't get into the mitochondria and be transformed into energy (for example: palmitic acid, which makes up 50% of the fat in food)*
- *L-carnitine helps increase the burning of fat under certain circumstances*
- *L-carnitine stimulates the burning of short-chain and medium-chain fatty acids (CoA)*
- *L-carnitine is necessary for the supply and production of energy*
- *L-carnitine helps to detoxifiy cells/mitochondria and optimizes cell metabolism*
- *L-carnitine helps to protect cell membranes against destruction by acids*
- *L-carnitine stories residual acetyl/acyl as quickly available energy*
  - ➤ *Helps to shorten recovery phase, increases protein synthesis*
  - ➤ *Supplier of acetate for syntheses such as acetylcholine from choline*
- *L-carnitine improves the course of all metabolic processes in which CoA participates, as well as glucose metabolism and protein metabolism*

In this type of diet, the supernutrient L-carnitine can also help prevent fatigue and exhaustion. According to nutrition experts, at least one and a half gram a day is the appropriate dosage for this purpose. As applies to fasting, additional doses of L-carnitine may tend to maintain the musculature while simultaneously improving the cell metabolism and reducing the fat reserves. Protection against the metabolic toxin ammonia is an important additional benefit.

Incidentally, L-carnitine helps maintain the blood-sugar level, avoiding the occurrence of low blood sugar. This helps to reduce the annoying sensation of hunger. If you have less hunger pangs, it is easier for you to diet successfully.

Anyone who eats lesser quantities of meat should take more L-carnitine.

Consumers have reported that L-carnitine sometimes reduces the sensation of hunger.

Areas Where L-Carnitine May Be of Potential Benefit

Aciduria	Distal ulcerative colitis	Myxedema
Adrenal insufficiency	Duchenne's dystrophy	Old age
AIDS	(pseudohypertrophic	Operations
Alcoholism	muscular dystrophy)	Overweight
Alzheimer's disease	Dysrhythmia	Ovo-lacto vegetarians
Anemia of the blood	Endurance sports	Peripheral circulatory
Angina pectoris	Epilepsy	disturbances
Artificial feeding	Extreme athletics	Pivampicillin therapy
Atherosclerosis	Fertility disorders	Post-polio symptoms (late
Avoidance of animal foods	Fitness training	sequelae)
Bechterew'sdisease (spondylitis	Heart attack	Pregnancy
deformans)	Heart diseases	Renal Fanconi's syndrome
Cancer	Heart failure	Renal insufficiency
Chemotherapy	Hyperammonemia	Reye's syndrome
Chronic Fatigue Syndrome (CFS)	Hyperthyroidism	Scleroderma
Chronic kidney disease	Hypertriglyceridemia	Sepsis
Chronic muscle myopathy	Hypoglycemia	Shock
Cirrhosis	Hypopituitarism	Smoker's leg
Competitive sports	Immune deficiency	Sperm
Connective tissue diseases	Intermittent Claudication	Stress
Dementia	(Charcot's Syndrome)	Stroke
Diabetes mellitus	Lactation and childhood	Tuberculosis
Dialysis	growth	Valproic-acid therapy
Diet lacking in carnitine	Liver disease	Varicose ulcers
Dieting	Muscle atrophy	Vegans
Diphtheria	Myocarditis	Vegetarians

L-Carnitine and Aerobic Training: The Power Team for Figure-Conscious People

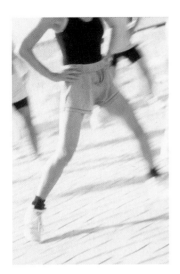

Aerobics—the ideal companion for L-carnitine when losing weight.

Anaerobic training leads to sore muscles and strains the metabolism.

Aerobic training deepens the breathing and promotes circulation.

L-carnitine can provide optimal support for a weight-management program if you simultaneously participate in aerobic training on a regular basis: During an aerobic workout, do the exercises for at least 30 minutes at such a light intensity that you don't have to "catch up" with your breathing when you stop.

We are all familiar with this: If we have to lift something heavy, perhaps while moving furniture. When we put it down our breathing continues to be deep and fast for a while. Why is this? The body had to mobilize more energy for the exertion than was possible with its available supply of oxygen. So it becomes necessary to supply the cells with oxygen again as quickly as possible afterward. This situation is called anaerobic training. When this kind of exertion is experienced over a longer period of time, the organism must take different paths that are completely independent of the direct supply of oxygen. But this solution isn't very healthy. Among other things, lactic acid is then produced, which can lead to sore muscles and increased wear of the tissue. Not to even mention the unpleasant pain involved. Afterward, the body must break down the lactic acid with a high expenditure of energy.

The situation is completely different for aerobic training. Through an even, long-term exertion that is still far below the limits of the highest performance level, the organism is stimulated to deepened breathing and improved circulation. Incidentally, fat is also broken down much better in this performance range than through a training program that turns the person into an exhausted and gasping candidate for sore muscles afterward.

If L-carnitine is used as a dietary supplement, considerably greater amounts of fat can be burned. Practiced on a regular basis, aerobic training has the effect of an oxygen treatment. The distinguished German physician Dr. Ernst van Aaken has used these types of physical exercise as a very effective supportive therapy for many chronic illnesses like cancer and Multiple Sclerosis.

Incidentally, since the middle of the 1980s, weight-management treatments at special clinics in the USA have been supported with megadoses of L-carnitine. Between 2 and 6 grams of the substance are given daily in many small portions to make losing weight through a weight management diet and a balanced exercise program more effective, healthier, and less stressful. According to the reports that I have seen about these programs, their success has been quite impressive.

I would like to emphasize one thing here: L-carnitine is not a diet pill in itself. However, it will help you manage weight in a better way and stay fit while doing so. But you must eat the proper diet and follow a fitness program as well.

Conclusion: You can manage your weight in an effective, healthy, and less stressful way with the help of L-carnitine.

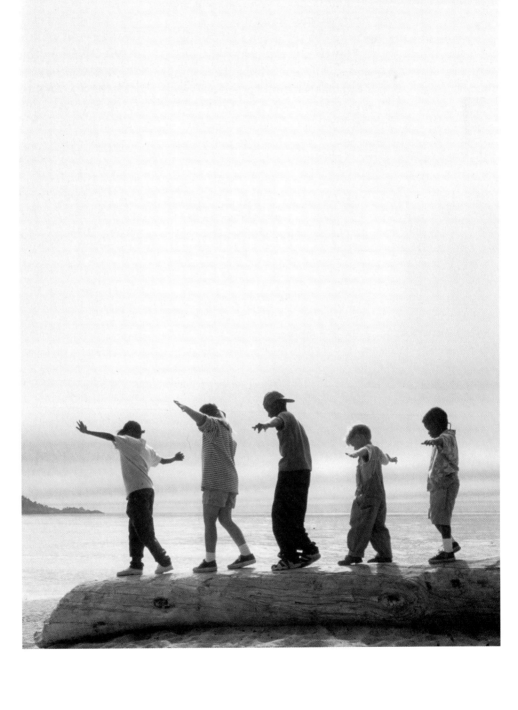

Chapter 3

Children and L-Carnitine: An "Essential" Topic

Children in particular need to be supplied with L-carnitine through food since their metabolism still has considerably less capacities for producing this substance than an adult's does. Only about twelve percent of the amount of L-carnitine that can be maximally synthesized in the fully developed human body is produced within a child's body. This means just a little more than one percent of the overall requirement! In the case of infectious diseases like the flu, colds, or various childhood diseases, or even an above-average amount of physical strain (like regular training on the soccer team or intensive play) drastically increases the metabolism's need for L-carnitine. The supply of L-carnitine through food becomes even more important.

Because of the minimal L-carnitine levels produced by their own bodies, active children in particular require an extra supply of this important substance.

In the case of milk allergies or analogous hypersensitivity, L-carnitine as a dietary supplement is a "must" for small children according to the opinion of leading nutritional specialists. By nature, a plant-based milk substitute contains practically no L-carnitine—except if the manufacturer is informed on this topic and has additionally supplemented the milk substitute with this vital substance that is essential for small children. Without L-carnitine, important functions in the organism are obstructed. Various studies have shown that an increased tendency toward illness, a reduction of vitality, and even growth disorders may occur.

Increase of Fertility

From the bottom of their hearts, many couples wish for children. Yet, their longing unfortunately often remains unfulfilled. In many of these cases, L-carnitine can help the dream of a family come true: When L-carnitine is supplied as a dietary supplement, the male sperm distinctly increase in vitality. As a result, the activity of the sperm is enhanced, as well as the number of sperm cells and fertility itself. The vitamin-like substance helps sperm produce energy.

Why?

L-carnitine provides the body with strength and promotes the production of healthy sperm cells. If it is lacking, the metabolism reduces the functions that are not necessarily vital for life in order to maintain the most important processes for securing immediate survival as well as possible. These functions include the production of fertile sperm. Mother Nature is actually quite clever in taking this precautionary measure. Used as a course of treatment, L-carnitine comprehensively promotes vitality. And as a natural consequence, the organism subsequently boosts the procreative capacity and directs more energy into increasing fertility.

Pregnancy

Because of mobilizing the reserves for the growth of the embryo, the mother's L-carnitine reserves are reduced. The cause of this is based not only on the higher requirements, but also in the frequently occurring iron deficiency, which also restricts L-carnitine production in the metabolism. A diminished ability to deal with strain on the physical and psychological level and an increased tendency toward infection may be the result. If L-carnitine is used as a dietary supplement, these unpleasant accompanying circumstances can be considerably improved. Since L-carnitine, as already discussed extensively above, strengthens and supplies additional energy reserves in a natural way, the birth may also be easier for the mother to endure and recover from more quickly.

When pregnant women have an iron deficiency, the production of L-carnitine is restricted.

The birth can be easier to endure and the mother can recover more quickly.

L-carnitine may particularly be meaningful as a dietary supplement for women with multiple or high-risk pregnancies.

According to the opinions of some nutritional experts, because of the virtually nonexistent supply of L-carnitine through the diet, pregnant vegetarians should definitely take this vitamin-like substance as a dietary supplement.

Premature Births

An adequate amount of L-carnitine strengthens the heart-and-lung function. This makes it an aid in helping "preemies" to better cope with their premature entrance into this world. Related studies clearly prove that premature babies have much better chances of survival with the appropriate dosage of L-carnitine. In addition, an appropriate L-carnitine level supports the lung maturation of the fetus.

Sudden Infant Death Syndrome (SIDS)

Most parents are probably haunted by the nightmare that their beloved child could become the victim of SIDS. There are indications that L-carnitine, already taken during pregnancy, may be protection against this terrible danger because of its vitalizing effect and strengthening of the child's lung and cardiovascular functions.

Strengthening the vital life functions can serve as protection against SIDS.

Breastfeeding

The mother's milk stays nutritious longer and the infant develops strong lung and heart functions more quickly.

People generally know that a breastfed child not only feels happier but is also given more robust health on its path in life. Although this is a wonderful time for the mother, it is also very strenuous and uses up much of her strength. In addition to healthy food and the additional dose of vitamins, minerals, and trace elements, L-carnitine can give the breastfeeding mother the energy reserves that help her enjoy the natural closeness with her child in this vital situation. Furthermore, it is a fact that when the mother is appropriately supplied with nutritional supplements her milk is nutritious for a much longer time. This naturally offers the child a much better supply of nutrients. On the other hand, if the mother's L-carnitine level is too low, she might have too little milk. Adequate amounts of L-carnitine in the milk also help the infant when strong lung and heart functions do not develop quickly enough.

Incidentally, if a breastfeeding mother decides upon a meat-free diet during the lactation period and if her infant is to be raised vegetarian, L-carnitine definitely should be taken as a dietary supplement. Otherwise, deficiencies and their corresponding health disorders will occur.

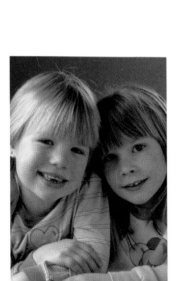

The strains of school stress can be reduced.

Schoolchildren

In some cases, memory and the ability to concentrate, verbal fluency, and mental capacity can be improved through L-carnitine. Children have problems adapting to the stress and strain of the school system, which has increased enormously in recent years. Taking L-carnitine naturally doesn't take the place of studying. However, it does make a tremendous difference when the mind is alert and clear and the child experiences a desire to learn instead of frustration.

Growth Disorders

In Switzerland and Italy, doctors prescribe up to 5 grams of L-carnitine per day as a well-tolerated, effective therapy for children with growth disorders.

In Switzerland and Italy, doctors prescribe up to 5 grams of L-carnitine per day as a well-tolerated, effective therapy for children with growth disorders. Since children cannot produce L-carnitine on their own, they are completely dependent upon having this vital substance supplied by their food. When adequate amounts of L-carnitine are not available because of a one-sided diet, it becomes difficult to maintain some of the metabolic functions. As a result, the child's normal growth is hindered. Without L-carnitine, for example, it is no longer possible to obtain energy by burning fats; consequently, the energy for the bodily functions is acquired by burning proteins and carbohydrates.

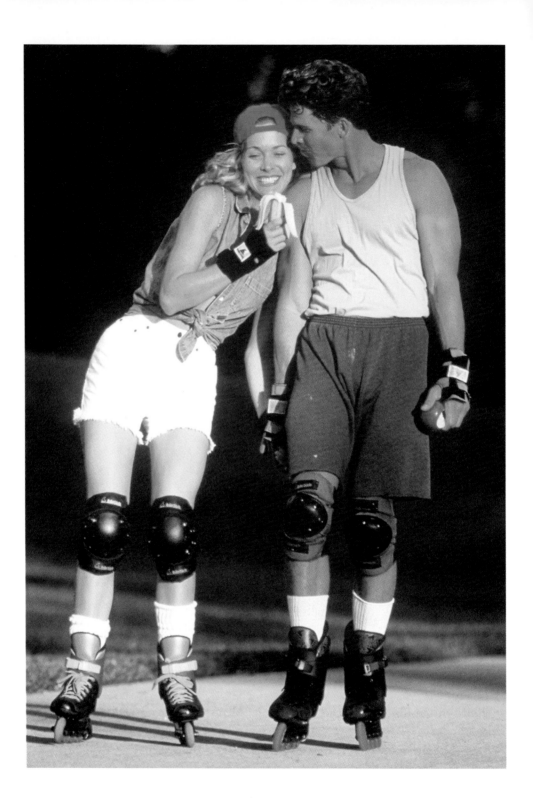

Chapter 4

L-Carnitine Wakes up Tired Athletes

Anyone who has had some experience with recreational sports is sure to be familiar with this situation: You start training to be really fit and perhaps even a bit slimmer for the summer swimming season. But first you have to put up with many days of sore muscles. And the feeling of vitality and resilience doesn't develop all that quickly after your training either. To the contrary: Most people usually tend to experience a feeling of low energy the day following an exercise session. And when you are finished with a training session, a feeling of ravenous hunger usually arises. A lot of willpower, idealism, and devotion to "self-torment" must be mobilized for the "trial training" to turn into a regular event. If you would like to work out successfully in a simpler and considerably more pleasant manner, then experiment with L-carnitine. Even during the 1980s, top athletes in almost every area used it with great success. Incidentally: Although L-carnitine, as a dietary supplement, can increase athletic performance, it isn't on the list of doping agents. After all, it is a substance that naturally occurs in the human body, which is also beneficial for overall health.

In relation to athletic training, the effects of L-carnitine speak for themselves:

➤ Drastic reduction of **sore muscles**
➤ Interception of the **toxin ammonia**, which is produced in the metabolism through the intensive physical strain, L-carnitine reduces the production of ammonia and improves its detoxification
➤ Short-term increase of the **muscle performance** up to about one-third, particularly for athletes who are less trained
➤ Less tendency toward injury (when taken on a regular basis in the individually appropriate amount, which should be determined by an experienced sports physician in case of doubt.)
➤ **Helps to stabilize the psyche**, even during high levels of strain and changing stress situations
➤ Clearly shortened recovery times after an intensive phase of **physical strain**

Also see Chapter 2, on pages 25 ff.

A great deal of willpower and idealism must be mobilized for "normal" training without L-carnitine.

Although L-carnitine, as a dietary supplement, can increase athletic performance, it isn't on the list of doping agents.

Also see The Secret of Success, on page 67. An interview with the holder of the overall world record in the Quintuple Ironman Triathlon.

Every athlete should include L-carnitine in his or her training program.

➤ Overall increase of **latent vitality**

➤ Helps to reducte susceptibility to infections, particularly during long-term **intensive training** periods

➤ Increase of **endurance and final-spurt performance.** Prevention of performance slumps after 70 to 90 minutes when the appropriate amount of L-carnitine is taken.

➤ **Reduced heart rate** (lower pulse rate) during physical strain, meaning that the heart performs at the same level with fewer beats.

➤ Release of stress enzymes is reduced

➤ Compensation for the considerable loss of L-carnitine during endurance sports. A runner loses up to two grams of L-carnitine over the marathon distance!

➤ The **training effect** on the musculature can be more intensive. The muscles not only can become stronger with supplementary L-carnitine but also can grow and show much more definition.

Effects of L-Carnitine in Sports (II)

- *L-carnitine helps to reduce premature tiring and mental exhaustion*
  - ➤ *Reduces the formation and effects of ammonia*
  - ➤ *Can lead to euphoric states, endorphins are more effective*
  - ➤ *L-carnitine and acetyl-carnitine have positive effects on brain/nerves*
  - ➤ *Strengthens concentration, increases mental capacity*
- *L-carnitine helps to improve muscle strength, muscle growth, and muscle transformation*
  - ➤ *Less risk of a mechanical strain*
  - ➤ *Increased protection against sore muscles, muscle-fiber tears, etc.*
  - ➤ *Type-1 fibers are increasingly formed (work aerobically afterward)*
- *Amino-acid pool (above all, BCAAs) may be spared*
  - ➤ *Less ammonia and urea is produced*
  - ➤ *After the training/competition, more amino acids may be available for protein synthesis and building up muscles*
  - ➤ *Increased anabolism, reduced catabolism, better training effect*

➤ **Circulation** and **respiration**, as well as the oxygen supply to the tissue, is clearly improved.

➤ The **life span** and number of red blood cells increases

➤ The **supply of blood to the legs** can be increased more than 8%

➤ A **more effective energy yield** for glucose utilization. Important for all short-term, high-level strains such as the sprint or track-and-field events

➤ Increase of the maximal **oxygen uptake, VO_2 max**, by up to 6%. This value is the average achieved in an experiment by the Italian sports physician *Marconi*, who had his test subjects take four grams of L-carnitine daily during a two-week period.

➤ Less frequent occurrence of stitches in the side through improvement of the **diaphragm function**.

➤ Buffering of harmful acids in the metabolism, which are often increasingly formed by a protein- and sugar-rich diet.

Experiments prove the effectiveness of L-carnitine.

- *Protein-rich diet helps to lower kidney performance, increases loss of L-carnitine*
- *Diminished performance, increased requirement must be compensated for*
- *L-carnitine helps to improve the circulation, respiration, and oxygen metabolism*
- *L-carnitine increases the life span and number of erythrocytes*
- *$VO2_{max}$ can be increased by 6 to11%*
- *L-carnitine increases the blood supply to the legs in athletes by 8.4%*
- *L-carnitine supports the diaphragm function and therefore the abdominal breathing*
- *L-carnitine helps to improve glucose utilization in the anaerobic phase*
- *May improve the energy yield for sprinters, for example*
- *Helps to improve and stabilize the immune system (open window)*
- *Protection against overstimulation and overstrain of the immune system*
- *80% of cases of death in sports are caused by myocarditis (athletes are 10 times more receptive to the Coxsackie virus than non-athletes)*
- *L-carnitine helps the heart in myocarditis*

Stimulates production of red blood cells to replace those destroyed during training.

➤ The production of red blood cells is stimulated: This is important because red blood cells are increasingly destroyed through intensive mechanical strain during training and competition. This is why athletes frequently suffer from a deficiency of vitamin B_{12}, B_6, and iron. The result is a restriction of the endogenous (body's own) L-carnitine synthesis.

"This simply sounds too good to be true!" is what you may now be thinking. But it can all be proved by the corresponding studies and reports on experiences, leaving absolutely nothing concealed in any kind of mystic fog. If you would like to do some research on your own, use the bibliography in the appendix.

What Is the Best Way to Use L-Carnitine for Sports?

➤ The window of the maximal increase in performance through L-carnitine is between two and six hours after taking it. So use L-carnitine at latest two hours before the start of training or competition.

➤ Since L-carnitine is difficult for the digestive tract to absorb when it occurs together with large amounts of amino acids, don't consume any protein drinks at the same time.

➤ Using L-carnitine on a regular basis is much more effective than taking it once before training since the L-carnitine reserves are only built up when taken over a longer period of time. In this way, the training effect can be put to optimal use.

➤ L-carnitine capsules, which dissolve in the small intestine, are the most suitable way of taking it.

➤ There is no legal limit assigned in the USA regarding the daily dosages of additional L-carnitine per day. If you would like to experiment with large doses, consult a physician experienced in nutritional issues for athletes before you begin using it.

For optimal effectiveness, a few rules must be observed.

Incidentally: During the World Soccer Championship in Spain in 1982, every member of the Italian team took L-carnitine during the event, which lasted six weeks. The teams of the other nations had not yet included this dietary supplement in their dietary programs. Of all the teams, the Italian players not only had the lowest injury rate, but also proved to have the best physical fitness on average—and became the world champions.

World Soccer Champions thanks to L-carnitine?

An interesting combination is L-carnitine with nutritional supplements like selenium, CO Q10, magnesium, vitamin C, vitamin-B complex, and vitamin E!

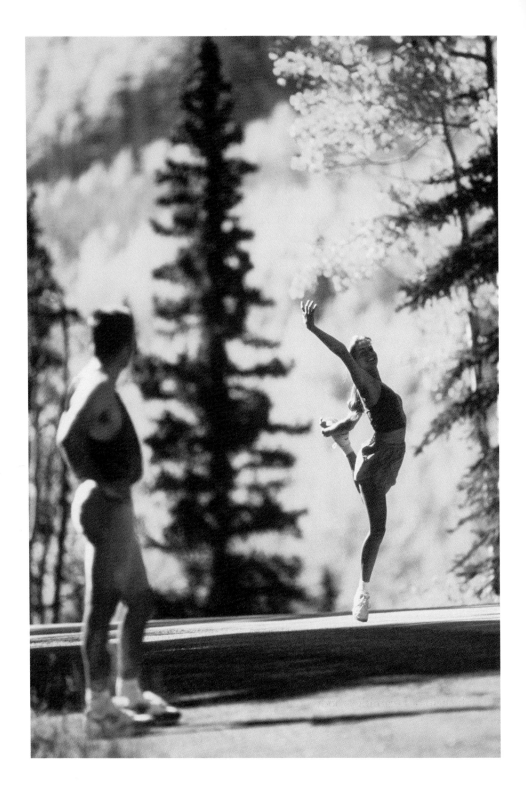

Chapter 5

L-Carnitine as a Fountain of Youth

The population of the Western industrial nations has a constantly increasing life span. However, despite improved medical care, this still doesn't mean that each individual also has a good quality of life. To the contrary—many chronic illnesses and diseases of attrition are on the advance and mar the well-earned golden age of life for some individuals. In my opinion, it isn't natural to become sicker and sicker in old age until death finally releases the person who has long been wasting away. Leading representatives of modern geriatrics believe that it currently is less important to intensively work on medical methods of additionally extending life span. Instead, efforts should be concentrated on raising the fundamental state of health and vitality in old age—and, consequently, the quality of life.

Enjoy your senior years —with health, vitality, and the highest quality of life.

Regeneration

L-carnitine, the jack-of-all-trades, is also capable of making a contribution in this situation. For example, the vitamin-like substance can help to slow down the aging process of the cells and even partially restore the damaged structure. A course of treatment with L-carnitine can therefore help to initiate extensive revitalization. Since the above-mentioned effects of L-carnitine are also directed at the nerve cells in particular, many of the disorders of the nervous system caused by aging can possibly ameliorated or effectively countered. In this context, I think it is important to mention the outstanding results of clinical experiments related to the suitability of L-carnitine in the management of symptoms of Alzheimer's disease, as well as slowing down the development of this terrible affliction.

Amelioration of nervous-system disorders caused by aging.

Physically Fit in Your Senior Years

With the help of L-carnitine, body strength and general physical capacity can not only be stabilized but also increased; this particularly applies when an individual uses a training and nutrition program developed especially for the respective age and condition of the person. In addition to specialists for geriatrics and some sport physicians, today many fitness clubs with well-trained employees also offer this kind of assistance in helping yourself. Since L-carnitine effectively reduces the unpleasant accompanying symptoms of working out and strengthens the exercise tolerance of the heart and lungs, many experts consider it to be virtually ideal for supporting a fitness program for the older generation. Between the 40th and the 80th year of life, up to 40% of the muscle mass is lost due to aging. Although the body weight may remain stable if an individual pays attention to diet and appropriate exercise, more fat is deposited because of the metabolism's reduced ability to burn fat. This not only promotes health disorders like the fatty degeneration of the heart muscle, fatty liver, arteriosclerosis, stroke, and muscle weakness, but can also be the cause of an increased requirement for L-carnitine with advancing age.

Effectively helps to reduce the unpleasant accompanying symptoms of training.

Mentally Alert and Active as a Senior

Many seniors are more afraid of no longer having clear minds than they are of coming down with a physical affliction. L-carnitine, with its positive effects on this problem, is a well-tolerated, very low-risk aid in this situation. It promotes mental functions in general, as well as fluency of speech, memory, and concentration in particular. In addition: A person who has vitality can more actively participate in life in every way. And this contribution toward maintaining mental capacity and mobility should not be underestimated. There's a good reason why "if you don't use it, you'll lose it."

L-carnitine helps to maintain the mental capacity…

How to Outwit Geriatric Disorders

It is a well-known fact that the afflictions occurring in old age—such as strokes, heart attacks, heart failure, arteriosclerosis, or diabetes don't just "suddenly" occur; sometimes their roots extend back more than a decade. Consequently, a person who does something in due time to prevent this will have a much better chance of not letting such nightmares ruin the enjoyment of retirement. Since L-carnitine normalizes and stabilizes the metabolism on a broad basis, it is suited for avoiding geriatric disorders like hardly any other bioactive substance.

…and is helpful on the management of a variety of geriatric diseases.

46

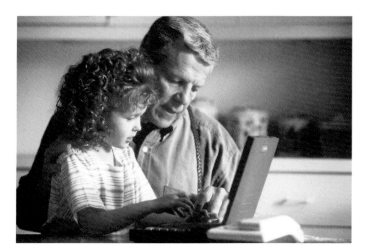

If such an affliction occurs prematurely, L-carnitine can often help subdue its development more than any similar substance. Diabetes, one of the most frequently occurring metabolic diseases of old age, can become considerably more manageable in its many symptoms through the additional administration of L-carnitine, for example.

L-Carnitine, or addition to improving fat metabolism also promotes healthy triglyceride and cholesterol levels.

To prevent the diseases of old age, many nutritional experts recommend working with daily doses of at least one gram. These should be distributed into two to four portions during a time period ranging from right after getting up to early afternoon, about 2 p.m. The capsules, which dissolve in the small intestine, are well-tolerated and particularly suited for this purpose. If it appears necessary to give higher doses in special cases, a healthcare practitioner with the appropriate training should be consulted.

L-carnitine helps to mantain healthy cholesteol and tryglyceride levels.

The well-tolerated capsules, which dissolve in the small intestine, are particularly good for taking controlled doses.

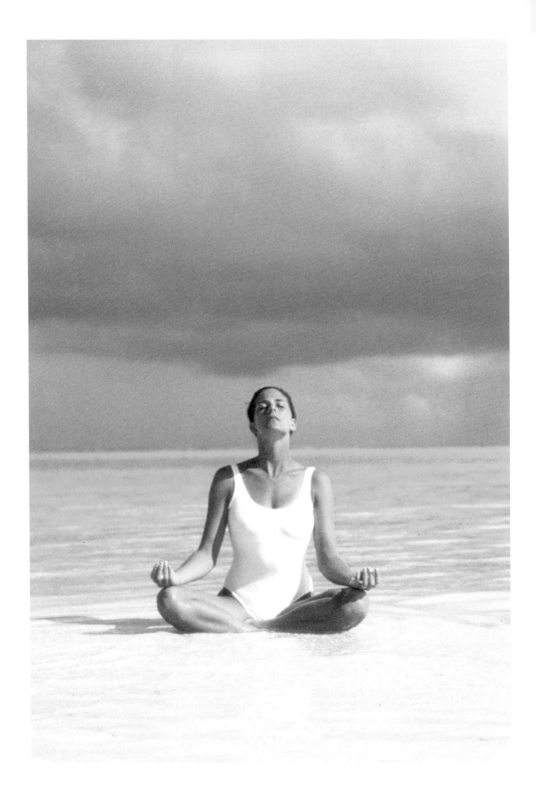

Chapter 6

How to Positively Influence Healing Processes with L-Carnitine

For an entire series of health disorders, L-carnitine can offer positive effects on vitality, the ability to regenerate, and the endogenous immune system. This chapter includes the most important areas for this application.

Within this context, here is one further note that may be useful for some people: If an examination determines a normal L-carnitine level in the blood serum and the person has one of the diseases listed here, these findings do not mean that giving additional L-carnitine as a dietary supplement would be superfluous. There may still be a so-called *relative* deficiency. This should be understood to mean that the existing amounts of the substance are not adequate for the body to overcome the metabolic problem. If a distinctly larger amount were to be available, it is often possible for normalization to be achieved.

"Normal" L-carnitine level versus relative L-carnitine deficiency.

AIDS

Acquired Immunodeficiency Syndrome (AIDS) is truly *the* epidemic of our age. After the infection, usually through sexual intercourse or a transfusion of contaminated blood, years often pass before the typical symptoms manifest themselves. In some people who are infected, the disease appears not to break out at all.

➤ Those suffering from AIDS get all kinds of secondary infections since their immune system is so weakened that the body is increasingly less capable of protecting itself against all types of contagion. Tumors, fungal infections, pneumonia, diarrhea, and many other problems literally make life hell. In this case, L-carnitine exercises a stabilizing influence.

➤ In addition, an increasingly intensive state of exhaustion occurs. Vitality diminishes more and more: accordingly, depressions occur more easily and the ability to enjoy life becomes increasingly limited. L-carnitine slows down the progress of the disease and mobilizes additional energies while simultaneously protecting the musculature. L-carnitine certainly isn't an AIDS remedy. Yet, corresponding reports on experiences in which test persons were given six grams of L-carnitine a day over a longer period of time show that this substance, which can be used in a variety of ways, may also help in these cases.

Optimizing the metabolic processes effectively supports the immune system.

➤ For example, L-carnitine effectively supports the immune system and supplies the urgently needed additional energy for fighting infections and tumor cells. This naturally only happens when the diet includes adequate calories. L-carnitine by itself isn't a fuel for the body. It only permits the important processes for gaining energy to run optimally or offers the preconditions for them to occur in the first place. The typical states of exhaustion can also be improved by means of L-carnitine.

➤ Some AIDS medications can cause side effects, including heart symptoms. L-carnitine can intervene here and extensively support the heart functions. (Also see the statements under the key word "Heart Diseases.") Since L-carnitine is frequently diminished in the metabolism of AIDS patients, it appears generally appropriate to examine whether taking this substance on a regular basis could be helpful.

➤ Studies in Italy, during which AIDS patients received up to six grams of L-carnitine as a dietary supplement for several weeks, showed distinctly positive results.

Alzheimer's Disease

In the industrial nations, this is the most frequently occurring form of pathogenic degeneration of the intellectual capabilities, such as memory. The causes of this terrible disease, which represent a difficult burden for the afflicted persons and their relatives, as well as society, have not yet been clarified.

During the years 1987 to 1989, patients suffering from Alzheimer's disease were supplemented with a dose of two grams of L-carnitine daily over a period of one year in clinical experiments in Italy. The study was carried out in the double-blind method and involved a control group, which was given a placebo. The evaluation showed astonishing results: The progress of the Alzheimer's symptoms was considerably delayed in the members of the group that had been given

L-carnitine! The exact therapeutic mechanism has not yet been explained. However, it appears that L-carnitine stabilizes the functions of the nerves and makes them, put into simple terms, less susceptible to damage through Alzheimer's disease. Further research in this regard is taking place throughout the world in order to clarify the opportunities that L-carnitine could offer people suffering from Alzheimer's disease.

We can expect to find even more positive effects on the nervous system.

The results of the Italian Alzheimer study are not surprising when we consider that other sources have shown that L-carnitine is involved with the formation of energy reserves for the brain: The aging process in the central nervous system can be slowed down, the memory and motor abilities may be improved, the nerves may be protected against various kinds of damage, and support is provided in healing damaged nerves.

Cancer

The immune system is generally weakened in the case of cancerous diseases. In addition, the cancer cells virtually "eat away" at the body. They draw a large portion of the energy-suppliers to themselves. As a result, the afflicted person suffers from increased weakening. In such cases, L-carnitine has two beneficial effects to offer: on the one hand, it supports the functioning of the immune system. On the other hand, it helps in providing energy. It is naturally important to supply enough calories through the diet so that the body's reserves are not further depleted. All things considered, it builds up the afflicted person and helps to provide the body with additional strength to fight against the cancer.

Furthermore, L-carnitine can help with certain harmful side effects of the currently applied chemotherapeutical agents on organs like the heart, as well as protecting the liver. This vitamin-like substance, helps to preserve cells against infections through tumors and also in some cases help protect from damage resulting from the poisonous chemotherapeutical agents.

The harmful side effects of chemotherapy can be alleviated.

Chronic Fatigue Syndrome (CFS)

In the case of CFS, the immune cells (macrophages) contain only about one-tenth of the normal amount of L-carnitine, strongly reducing the functional capacity of the body's own defense system. The symptoms of CFS can be relieved through L-carnitine.

51

Diabetes

The organism of diabetics produces toxic ketones, which are also responsible for typical "bad breath". It has been known since the mid-1970s that L-carnitine is capable of facilitating the burning of ketones, whereby they can increasingly be rendered harmless. In addition, it also reduces the formation of these harmful substances.

The tolerability of sugar, also called the glucose-tolerance factor in medical jargon, can be distinctly improved by L-carnitine. The result is that sugar values in the blood are not as high.

Diabetes is considered to be a *metabolic disease*. Consequently, keeping the blood-sugar values at as much of a normal value as possible by administering insulin may be inadequate as the correct treatment. Diabetics also have a disturbed fat metabolism. Fats are increasingly mobilized as energy bearers for the cells that are suffering from starvation, but because of a relative deficiency of L-carnitine, they cannot be burned in appropriate amounts. With time, this easily leads to damaging the cardiovascular system and increased risk of stroke. As described under the key word "Heart Diseases," the dietary supplement L-carnitine can be especially valuable here in keeping the heart healthy and efficient. Diabetics eliminate much more L-carnitine than healthy people do, so even this fact indicates that it may be wise to give them extra doses of L-carnitine. A major problem for people who have been suffering from diabetes for a longer period of time is the deteriorated wound healing. Since L-carnitine supports the circulation and the immune system, as well as stimulating the oxygen supply to cells, it can also help counter these symptoms.

For diabetics, both the fat metabolism and the healing of wounds are improved.

Heart Diseases

The heart is the most important place for the effects of L-carnitine. No wonder that it has a potential beneficial influence on all heart disorders based on metabolic reasons. Among other things, there are promising reports on:

Positive effects on many heart diseases.

➤ **Cardiomyopathy** (heart-muscle disease). One of the most frequent indications for heart transplants and cause of death for 80% of all young athletes is, the development of this heart disease, which is caused by viruses. L-Carnitine helps to increase the chances of survival and reduces the number of necessary heart pacemaker transplants.

➤ **Heart attack.** When there is an oxygen deficiency in the heart musculature, fatty acids are no longer burned. In turn, this blocks the heart function. In this case, L-carnitine provides for the normalization of fat metabolism in the heart. It consequently is important in an infarction situation.

➤ **Angina pectoris.** Pain-free periods are lengthened. The ability to tolerate exercise and without pain is increased.

➤ **Additional therapies for heart attack.** It has now been clinically demonstrated that L-carnitine reduces the extent of a heart attack and accordingly increases survival chances for the afflicted individual.

➤ **Weakness of the heart muscle.** L-carnitine helps to strenghten the heart and improves the functional capacity by increasing energy production.

Fatty acids cover 80% of the heart's energy requirements!

➤ **Cardiac dysrhythmia** (disorders of the heart rhythm). L-carnitine exercises a normalizing influence on existing disorders.

➤ **Fatty degeneration of the heart muscle.** L-carnitine helps to increase the burning of fat and therby it helps to avoid blocking of the heart functions.

Why Do Heart Diseases Respond So Well to L-Carnitine?

The heart musculature needs fatty acids as a supply of energy. Consequently, it needs them to maintain the constant, vitally important pumping action that moves the blood through the body. Fatty acids are the essential energy-suppliers for the heart. L-carnitine is particularly important for this purpose since it transports the fatty acids into the mitochondria, the biological powerhouses inside the cells. A heart muscle that is well nourished is less likely to become ill. It is better at dealing with strain and recovers more quickly. It has also been observed that athletes taking L-carnitine on a regular basis have the same training performance at a reduced number of heartbeats (slower pulse). Accordingly, the heart is potentially subject to less strain only when the organism has sufficient L-carnitine available to it.

Fatty acids improve the energy supply for the heart muscle.

According to studies by the research institute in Juelich, Germany, heart attacks are preceded by a serious disorder of the regulated fat-burning process. As a result, fatty acids can collect in the heart tissue, for example, and contribute to a deteriorating disposal of the waste materials and toxins in the area, as well as a reduced supply with nutrients. L-carnitine has a normalizing effect in this case. It can even help repair damage to a certain extent.

Since the heart is the organ in the body that contains the most L-carnitine of all, it is basically no wonder that additional amounts of L-carnitine are so good at supporting this vital organ.

In somewhat simplified terms, the autoimmunological processes that lead to damage of the heart muscle are triggered by damage to the normal fat metabolism in the situation of cardiomyopathy.

In autoimmunological diseases, the endogenous (body's own) immune system attacks portions of its own organism. It no longer recognizes the difference between pathogenic intruders like bacteria, viruses, or fungal spores and the cells of its own body.

When heart patients are treated with L-carnitine, the effectiveness of the treatment appears to be increased when an additional ample supply of vitamin B_1 (thiamin) is also given.

Hypoglycemia

Hypoglycemia (low blood sugar) has been often noticed as the first sign of an L-carnitine deficiency, resulting in symptoms like depression, fatigue, and carbohydrate cravings. Supplementation with L-carnitine is advised since it helps the liver to burn fat and produce the glucose required to stabilize the blood sugar levels. If untreated, hypoglycemia can lead to progressive muscular disorders, heart tissue damage, poor brain functioning, and diabetes.

Infectious Diseases

The immune system needs a great deal of energy in order to fulfill its functions—the destruction of the germs that invade the body and neutralization of toxins and waste substances For example, the macrophages can move independently within the organism. However, this also requires a great deal of energy. If the immune system turns up to full speed because of an infection, much of the reserves of L-carnitine are drawn off to supply it. This is like a general mobilization in the case of war, where a large portion of the country's resources is also made available to the military so that it can fulfill its tasks.

The macrophages contain twenty times as much L-carnitine as the blood plasma surrounding them and are therefore dependent upon an adequate supply of the vitamin-like substance.

In such a case, L-carnitine is at risk of being in short supply for other tasks of the metabolism, such as the energy supply for the musculature. Exhaustion, increased fatigue, and a reduced ability to deal with psychological stress are potential consequences.

The traditional recipe for people who are lying in bed exhausted with a heavy cold is to cook a good beef broth or (chicken soup) so that they can get "back on their feet" again. It is possible that this well-known "remedy" is so effective because of the L-carnitine contained in the meat, which is quite soluble in water and therefore passes into the soup during cooking. Taken as a dietary supplement, L-carnitine can naturally help in a much better form. Between 300 mg and 1,000 mg daily, according to age and body weight, can contribute a great deal toward supporting the immune system enough so that it can resist infections. This may also help shorten the length of the illness. In addition, vitality is better maintained and the recuperation period (convalescence) may be shortened. The illness is not protracted as easily but cured in a natural way, as it should be. This naturally applies not only to flu infections but basically to all infectious diseases as well.

Beef broth—one of the oldest ways of giving L-carnitine.

Simultaneously, the activity and multiplication of the immune system's macrophages is increased. Since L-carnitine may also stimulate the production of antibodies, practically the entire endogenous defense system is positively influenced by it.

And don't worry: You can go ahead and experiment with L-carnitine because it isn't toxic. There has been no evidence of contraindications nor negative interactions with medications. Even when taking it over a longer period of time, it will cause damage or lead to an addictive effect.

Go ahead and experiment with the positive effects of L-carnitine.

Contrary to most of the plant-based immunostimulants with which I am familiar, L-carnitine can be taken in any phase of an infectious disease; including fever, no matter how high; chronic and acute infections; and even sepsis. But when you use it, please remember that it takes about two hours until L-carnitine is fully effective.

Intermittent Claudication (Charcot's Syndrome)

L-carnitine has been shown to improve the circulation of the legs: As a possible result, the person once again has more strength to walk and the pain tends to decrease. The vitamin-like substance promotes a better energy supply and waste disposal for the cells. It also promotes the oxygen-transport function through the increased formation of red blood cells. Since L-carnitine also helps to make more strength available on an

L-carnitine promotes increased stamina.

overall basis, it is no wonder that a considerably longer distance can often be walked without pain.

Liver Diseases

Since the endogenous synthesis of L-carnitine takes place in the liver, many diseases that affect the liver also equally damage the human organism's ability to supply itself with this substance. It is highly recommended that people in this situation take additional doses of L-carnitine as a dietary supplement since it also fundamentally offers positive effects in relation to the liver. L-Carnitine helps to protect its regeneration is promoted, and various important functions improved.

Muscle Atrophy

Since L-carnitine promotes the energy supply to the musculature, in many cases it is possible to delay the loss of vitality and improve the general state of health.

Operations

L-carnitine supports the functioning of the immune system. Consequently, the risk of infection after operations may be reduced. Furthermore, it helps to improve vitality and accelerate the convalescence period. The formation of blood cells is promoted, as well as the overall vital functions of the red blood cells. The risk of thrombosis may be lowered since L-carnitine helps to counteract the clumping of erythrocytes and improve the fluidity of the blood on a broad basis.

As a dietary supplement, L-carnitine is especially recommended for operations accompanied by the loss of large amounts of blood.

L-carnitine supports the formation of blood cells.

If blood is taken from a patient before an operation so that it isn't necessary to depend on blood donors in case of blood loss, L-carnitine can support the formation of blood cells and thereby helps to shorten the waiting period before the date of the operation.

Post-Polio Syndrome (Late Sequelae)

L-carnitine has also been shown to be very helpful for harmonizing the late sequelae of polio since it promotes strenghtening of the musculature and nervous system. Up to one gram of the substance daily as a dietary supplement on a long-term basis helps stabilize the muscle function and general well-being. If it appears appropriate to use larger daily doses in individual cases, consult a specialized healthcare practitioner for this purpose. Here is a summary of the effects:

➤ Tiredness is reduced

➤ Endurance is increased

➤ The recovery phases are shortened

Renal Insufficiency

When the kidneys can no longer adequately purify the blood of the substances that are usually eliminated with the urine, the body poisons itself with the metabolic residue. Today, in such cases a dialysis (washing the blood by means of an artificial kidney) is carried out on a regular basis. Every few days, a machine takes over the tasks of the weakened kidneys and purifies the blood. However, large amounts of L-carnitine are also removed from the blood in this process. Healthy kidneys hold back this vital substance. There is still no equipment that can compare with the human body's achievements. As explained in previous chapters, when there is an increased requirement the body's own L-carnitine synthesis cannot supply enough to guarantee the level required to maintain vitality. The limit is reached at about ten percent of the normal requirement. The customary supply through the diet also isn't necessarily adequate in such extreme cases. Additional doses of L-carnitine in the form of a dietary supplement can be helpful here. Consult the attending healthcare practitioner for an exact individual dosage.

L-carnitine is also "washed out" of the blood during dialysis.

Smoker's Leg and Varicose Ulcers

L-carnitine promotes circulation in the legs and promotes healing of leg ulcers. L-carnitine promotes circulation in the legs and improves the healing of ulcers on the legs. Because of the extensive positive effects of L-carnitine on the immune system, waste products are broken down more quickly and infections of all types are healed more easily. The formation of new cells is stimulated. Moreover, L-carnitine extends the life of the red blood cells and supports their function in the metabolism; in addition, it also improves the fluidity of the blood. This contributes to reducing the possibility of deposits in the blood veins.

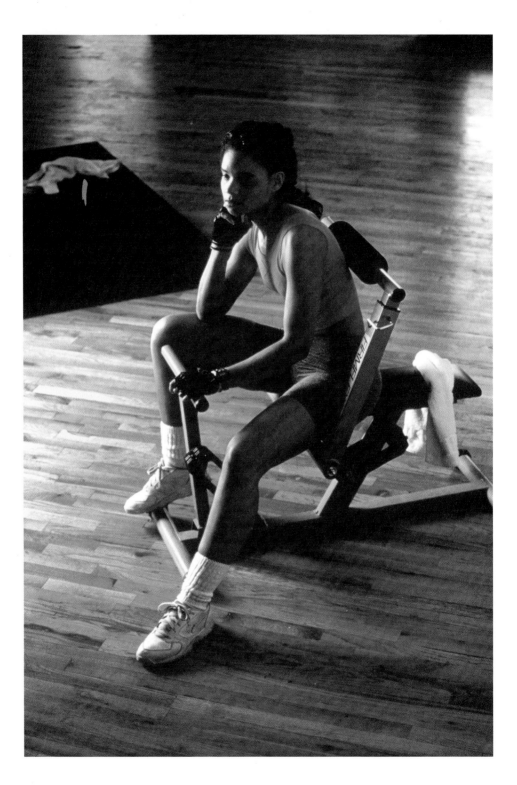

Chapter 7

Questions and Answers on the Topic of L-Carnitine

When L-Carnitine Is Manufactured, Isn't There a Risk of BSE (Bovine Spongiform Encephalopathy) Pathogens in the Dietary Supplement?

It's been a long time since meat has been used to manufacture L-carnitine for nutritional supplements. One major reason for this is because it would be totally uneconomical: The costs would be about 1,500(!) times higher than that of the bio-technological production. Accordingly, we can rule out that meat contaminated with BSE pathogens will land in the L-carnitine for nutritional supplements.

L-carnitine is not extracted from meat.

Is Genetic Technology Used in the Production Process?

The answer is very clear: **No!** L-carnitine is manufactured from naturally occurring raw materials through various chemical reactions and by the use of bacteria cultures that can be found everywhere in healthy soil (also see chart on next page). These "little helpers" metabolize certain source substances and produce L-carnitine. Described in broad terms, this last step in the manufacturing of L-carnitine is a process similar to how dough is treated in sourdough, sauerkraut is made, or grape juice is fermented into wine.

Isn't It Unnatural to Take Extra L-Carnitine?

L-carnitine occurs in the tissue of every animal. It is absolutely necessary for providing the supply of energy. Since the human body can only produce minor amounts of L-carnitine

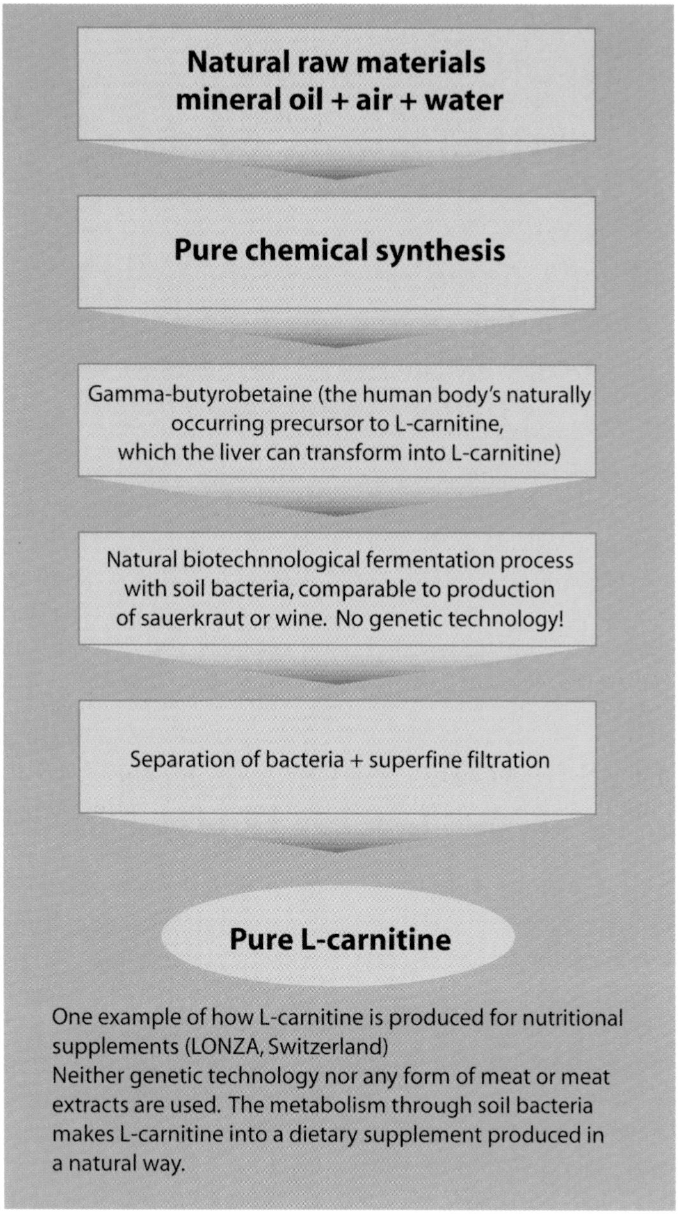

Natural raw materials
mineral oil + air + water

⬇

Pure chemical synthesis

⬇

Gamma-butyrobetaine (the human body's naturally
occurring precursor to L-carnitine,
which the liver can transform into L-carnitine)

⬇

Natural biotechnnological fermentation process
with soil bacteria, comparable to production
of sauerkraut or wine. No genetic technology!

⬇

Separation of bacteria + superfine filtration

⬇

Pure L-carnitine

One example of how L-carnitine is produced for nutritional
supplements (LONZA, Switzerland)
Neither genetic technology nor any form of meat or meat
extracts are used. The metabolism through soil bacteria
makes L-carnitine into a dietary supplement produced in
a natural way.

Manufacturing process for L-carnitine.

itself, and therefore can only meet a little more than ten percent of the average requirement—far short of the requirement for unusual strain!—the supplying of L-carnitine through the diet is absolutely necessary in order to be stress-resistant and healthy. Today, we are confronted with a multitude of unnatural and very stressful influences—such as chemicals in our food and the environment, increased exposure to radiation through electrical equipment (cell phones, monitors, power lines) of all types—while having developed an eating "culture" that destroys the important vital substances in the food and/or removes them during preparation. Consequently, many nutritional experts believe there is an increasing necessity for using certain bioactive substances like vitamin C or L-carnitine as nutritional supplements. People who eat a vegetarian diet, or even a vegan diet, get almost no L-carnitine through their food since this substance is only found in minor amounts in fruit, grain, vegetables, and nuts. Taking L-carnitine on a regular basis is very much recommended in this situation. Vegetarian expectant and breastfeeding mothers are strongly advised to use L-carnitine as a dietary supplement in order to avoid deficiency diseases and damage to organs, as well as helping to promote the normal growth of their children.

Vegans eat a diet consisting only of plant products. In contrast to vegetarians, they even do without dairy products and eggs.

Is L-Carnitine Toxic in Any Form?

No! This is an endogenous substance (made by the body itself), which naturally occurs in all of our bodies in quite large amounts—about 20 to 25 grams. As clearly demonstrated by clinical studies, even taking several grams of L-carnitine per day has no known toxic effects on the body.

Are There Side Effects When Taking L-Carnitine?

In rare cases, side effects have been observed when taking L-carnitine. At very high dosages, trembling and hyperactivity, problems in falling asleep, and diarrhea may occur. What "very high" means depends upon the body weight, training condition, and general state of health. However, this doesn't classify it as having a "toxic" effect. These side effects are simply based upon energy provided by the body that cannot be utilized at that moment. In case something like this happens because of unfortunate circumstances, an antidote has been recommended by someone who has experienced this situation: Keep calm until the excess L-carnitine has been eliminated through the urine. Drinking several glasses of water helps in this process. Howev-

In case of an "overdose," drink a lot of water.

er, individuals suffering from heart disease or nervous disorder should call a physician for safety's sake. The same applies when the symptoms do not immediately improve after resting.

However, people who currently have intensive physical strains to master will most likely not experience any of these side effects, even with ten grams of L-carnitine every day. There are reports of top athletes who take corresponding amounts of L-carnitine at competitions: They don't experience any problems with it and even achieve an enormous increase in performance, both physically and mentally.

Another side effect can occur when taking L-carnitine in powder form or as a liquid preparation on an empty stomach. On the one hand, nausea and vomiting may occur, especially at high dosages. On the other hand, there are some bacteria cultures in the intestines that metabolize L-carnitine. This can lead to flatulence and diarrhea. But please note: These symptoms do not occur for everyone. Incidentally, they are easy to prevent: Either take the L-carnitine together with a meal so it isn't quite as concentrated or take it in capsule form. Gelatin capsules don't dissolve until they reach the small intestine, so the corresponding bacteria have much less contact with the substance and there are no unpleasant accompanying symptoms.

Strictly speaking, L-carnitine has no harmful side effects in the sense of toxic effects or lasting functional disorders of the organs. Diarrhea and similar symptoms also occur when there is an overdose of vitamin C or the sweetener sorbitol, for example.

No contraindications have been discovered up to now.

Some bacteria "eat" L-carnitine and eliminate the remainder in a converted form.

The side effects are comparable to those of an overdose of vitamin C or sorbitol (sweetener).

Also see Monograph on page 73.

Are There Any Known Intolerances or Allergies?

Fundamentally, there can be allergies or intolerances to absolutely any substance. So the same applies to L-carnitine. However, according to my research, there have been no appreciable problems associated with this up to now.

Is It Habit-Forming?

There can be no habit-formation or addiction to L-carnitine since this substance exists in every healthy body in larger amounts and is constantly required for its healthy functioning. However: There is the "danger" of getting used to the above-average level of psychological and physical capacity and vitality that is promoted by taking an appropriate amount of L-carnitine on a regular basis and no longer wanting to miss this pleasant state.

Who Particularly Needs This Dietary Supplement?

In my opinion, this dietary supplement is for anyone who would like to be fit for today's everyday life with its practically unavoidable and mostly unnatural chemical, physical, and psychological strains.

Anyone can benefit from the positive effects!

But L-Carnitine is expecially recommended to the following: expectant mothers, small children, (fitness) athletes, smokers, people who have an above-average stress level in their professional or private lives, people suffering from a weakening disease like cancer or AIDS, and those who have health disorders that respond especially well to additional doses of L-carnitine.

Furthermore, experts highly recommend it in relation to operations that may be accompanied by losses of larger amounts of blood because it helps to promote the formation of red blood cells and strengthens the immune system.

Another area of use is for people who are quickly exhausted and all those who have weight problems.

Vegetarians and vegans will profit a great deal from L-carnitine as a dietary supplement since their diet makes very little or none of it available to them. Vegetarian expectant and breastfeeding mothers are stongly advised to take additional L-carnitine in order to avoid deficiencies and not endanger the healthy growth of their children.

Is L-Carnitine a Medication?

The answer varies from country to country. The word medication (from the Latin *medicamentum* = healing remedy) is used for everything made from natural raw materials or produced on a synthetic basis that is applied to diagnostic, therapeutic, or preventive application in relation to health. In comparison, nutrients are all the substances that the organism can use for producing its own components.

I'm not the only person who has difficulty in differentiating between nutritional/dietary supplements and medications once in a while. Some people have started using the term nutrication to describe foods that can have a healing effect. For example, the criteria for L-carnitine are similar to that for vitamin C. Because they contain an "overdose" of the vitamin, ripe pepper pods would have to be banned to the pharmacy as a vitamin-C medication. And what about water? Used in therapeutic doses, it has proved to heal or at least clearly improve some serious illnesses. However, we should naturally pay attention to any applicable government regulations.

This classification of L-carnitine does not exist in the USA. According to the *Dietary Supplement Health and Education Act* of 1994 (DSHEA) "A dietary supplement is a product intended to supplement the diet, containing a vitamin, mineral, herb of other botanical or amino acid, or a concentrate, metabolite, constituent, extract, of combination of such ingredients."

Does L-Carnitine Supplementation Harm the Body's Own Production of It?

In order to be optimally supplied, the body must receive L-carnitine from the outside.

No, it is completely normal for the human organism to have L-carnitine supplied to it through the diet. The L-carnitine used as a dietary supplement is not different than the form that occurs in nature. It is treated exactly like the L-carnitine in food by the metabolism.

In addition, the endogenous production of L-carnitine is a so-called enzymatic reaction. This basically cannot be damaged by the external supply of L-carnitine. The production of L-carnitine in metabolism is reduced when adequate amounts of the substance are absorbed into the body through the diet. If the supply from the outside is too limited, the organism once again regulates the synthesis of L-carnitine upwardly with a minor time delay. However, the amount of endogenous production of the vitamin-like substance is not increased above a value of about ten percent of the normal requirement. Then deficiency symptoms tend to occur. The only way that the body can help itself in this situation is by eliminating less L-carnitine through the kidneys than it does when there is an

64

ample supply of it. However, the system is designed so that 100% absorption never occurs. Consequently, the L-carnitine level in the body is still reduced, even if this occurs in a slow but continuous manner. When there is long-lasting physical strain, L-carnitine is also eliminated. For example, about two grams are eliminated during a marathon run!

Do Negative Interactions Occur?

According to my research, there are no known negative interactions with medications.

Also see Monograph on page 73.

However, under certain circumstances there may be a reduction in the absorption of L-carnitine from nutritional supplements when taken together with a larger amount of amino acids. An example of this is the protein drinks that are popular in the fitness arena. So it is recommended that you take L-carnitine at a different time to achieve an optimal effect. About one hour is recommended as the time interval between having a power drink and taking an L-carnitine preparation.

Do not take L-carnitine together with protein.

What Is the Proper Dosage for L-Carnitine?

Children can be given between 25 and 100 mg for each kilogram (2.2 pounds) of body weight orally, in several doses a day.

Adults can take up to 5 grams per day.

Should L-Carnitine Be Taken during Pregnancy and Breastfeeding?

Since this is an endogenous substance that isn't toxic and no contraindications are known, risks should not be expected in these cases. To the contrary—various research work and reports on experience from women in these situations permit the conclusion that L-carnitine taken by the mother during pregnancy and breastfeeding can greatly contribute to the well-being and health of both mother and child. Pregnant and breastfeeding vegetarian women are strongly advised to use L-carnitine as a dietary supplement to prevent deficiencies and promote the healthy growth of their children.

L-carnitine can contribute a great deal toward the well-being of pregnant and breastfeeding women.

Are There Negative Effects on Drivers and Machine-Operators?

Also see Monograph on page 73.

There are no known negative effects in these cases.

In What Forms Can It Be Taken?

L-carnitine is added to various fitness drinks and power bars. In addition, it can be purchased in the following forms:
• Tablets
• Lozenges
• Gelatin capsules (soluble in the small intestine)
• Powder
• Spray
• Syrup (with alcohol)
• Effervescent tablets
• Powder for preparing refreshment drinks
• Chewable tablets similar to gumdrops
• Ampoules for drinking

When Can L-Carnitine Help in Managing Weight?

When fitness training is engaged in at the same time, L-carnitine increases the extent of weight reduction.

When a person simultaneously engages in fitness training, L-carnitine increases the rate of weight reduction by more than ten percent. Yet, this is only a small portion of the way it promotes weight management. If we feel good and strong, we are more likely to work out, as well as doing it more frequently and intensively. L-carnitine can also help to reduce the unpleasant accompanying symptoms in the form of sore muscles, feelings of exhaustion, or ravenous hunger that can occur directly after training or even the next day. As a result, it has the effect of an all-round support in helping an individual slim down and stay that way. In a natural way, it also helps counter the feelings of reluctance, largely based on the metabolism, that generally occur during fasting or a weight-management diet. At least one gram a day should be taken for this purpose.

Appendix I

The Secret of Success

The overall world-record holder in the Quintuple Ironman Triathlon, Astrid Benohr, talks about her experiences with nutritional supplements and L-carnitine

An interview by
Dr. Stefan Siebrecht, B.S. in Biochemistry

Astrid Benohr (born on Oct. 8, 1957, height 1.66 meters, weight 50 kg) is the mother of three children and world record-holder in the Double, Triple, Quadruple, and Quintuple Ironman Triathlon. She was and is the first woman to hold an overall world record for men and women. Even the "man with most endurance in the world" requires two more hours, that means 76 hours, 16 minutes for a Quintuple Ironman Triathlon (19 km swimming, 900 km bicycling, 210 km running) than Astrid Benohr.

Two hours faster than the fastest man!

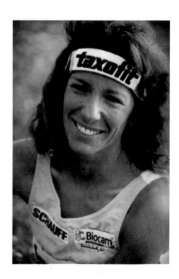

Ms. Benohr, even marathon runners think that your achievements are superhuman. Is there an explanation for your extreme endurance performance or can people be trained to do something like this?
"In my opinion, women are more capable of performing in the extreme endurance areas than men are. This is probably related to the different fat metabolism and the lower body weight of women. By comparison, the marathon run is a short distance in which the strength of men can still clearly dominate.

In addition, I have found the right balance between physical stress and regeneration. My special diet, which is adapted to the level of strain, is also one of the most important preconditions and absolutely necessary for me. My training time is actually quite short, about 20 to 30 hours a week. Moreover, I use many open cross-country races as training. However, before an ultra competition, I prescribe myself a seven-to-ten day forced break in order to gather my strength."

"Women are more capable of performing in the extreme endurance areas than men."

How often can you go through these depleting competitions every year?

"I participate in about 30 competitions per year, of which only six are the big ultra triathlons. It might be possible to do more, but the health risk is too high for me."

How do you eat during an ultra-triathlon competition?

> **The type of food and right point in time must be well-coordinated.**

"During the competition, I need to be supplied with an enormous amount of carbohydrates, proteins, minerals, vitamins, and other substances in an easily digestible form. The amount and point in time must also be coordinated in the process. Mineral drinks and energy bars have proved to be optimal for this purpose, but I've also tested bananas and even hamburgers. I've already tried out many nutritional tricks and have also had some bad experiences in the process."

With what kind of dietary approaches have you had bad experiences?

> **Decrease in performance through a high-carbohydrate vegetarian diet.**

"I once had a strict vegetarian diet for weeks and ate only a large amount of whole-grain products and muesli. As a result, my performance was less than satisfactory and I felt noticeably worse during the competition and afterward. At that point, I recognized that diet plays a decisive role in endurance sport and nutritional supplements are also important."

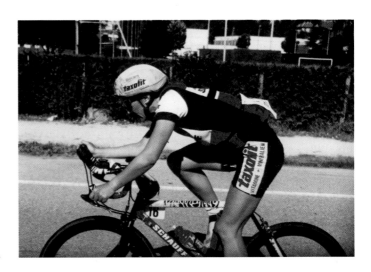

Astrid Benohr at a triathlon.

You've been doing the triathlon since 1984. It is conspicuous that your greatest successes were all after 1991. Is this related to the change in your diet and the use of nutritional supplements?

"Certainly, but not solely. An optimal diet and nutritional supplements are one of the many basic preconditions for being able to attain and repeat such a performance. But in order to set a new world record today, everything must be right. There are many additional factors involved."

When and how did you discover L-carnitine for yourself?

"It was in 1991, shortly before the first Double Triathlon in Lelystad (Netherlands). I actually ran my first world record right away there. At the time, I worked as an assistant for Professor Uhlenbruck in the Immunological Institute at the University of Cologne. Professor Uhlenbruck got me involved in running and also recommended that I take L-carnitine."

World record after taking L-carnitine.

What experiences have you had with L-carnitine since 1991?

Above all, I feel better with L-carnitine when regenerating and am back in shape more quickly. Since I train purely according to feeling, there is the danger that I feel "too good and fit" through L-carnitine and then participate again too soon. I therefore have to force myself to observe the regeneration period and be careful not to overestimate myself. In addition, my resistance to stress has increased since I've been taking L-carnitine. I'm noticeably better at coping with the competitions and regenerate more quickly. This reduction of stress was also illustrated by the test data. In July of 1997 at the Triple Triathlon in Lensahn (Germany), Professor Neumann from University of Düsseldor in Germany found that among all athletes, I had the lowest blood centrations of stress enzymes."

Stress is demonstrably reduced during competitions.

According to Professor Uhlenbruck, L-carnitine has a positive effect on the immune system. Have you noticed something of this effect in recent years?

"The fact is that since 1991, which means since I started taking L-carnitine, I've no longer needed any antibiotics and have been free of illnesses and injuries. This may be related to L-carnitine, but it doesn't have to be. It is probably difficult to pinpoint the cause and effect in this situation."

You've participated in the Quintuple Ironman twice and have run a world record each time. However, the second time you were 12.5 hours faster. What was different the second time?

"I ran the first Quintuple Ironman in 1994 in Den Haag (Netherlands) too soon after the Triple Triathlon in Fontanil (France). In Den Haag I managed to break the women's world record with 86 hours and 44 minutes, but two men were ahead of me. Furthermore, it was my first experience in the Quintuple Ironman and I was probably also somewhat weakened because of Fontanil beforehand. At the second attempt in September of 1997, I was able to profit from the experiences in Den Haag."

Is it true that you took megadoses of L-carnitine for the first time in 1997 in Kerpen, where you achieved the overall world record in the Quintuple Ironman Triathlon for the first time?

An optimal combination of L-carnitine, carbohydrates, and minerals gives a burst of energy.

"That actually wasn't intentional. Normally, I take 4 to 5 grams of L-carnitine per training week. However, during the competition I drank an entire jar of a mineral drink by Multipower. That was about 20 liters (quarts) of the drink divided over three days. The combination of the drink made of carbohydrates and minerals was really optimal. In addition, I took in 20 grams of L-carnitine with this drink, which means about seven grams per day. I was really surprised by the effect. During the competition, I felt astonishingly well and also recovered at an amazing speed afterward. This drink gave me the right burst of energy each time."

Ms. Benohr, thank you for the interesting conversation.

Appendix II

Why Should Nutritional Supplements Be Used at All?

by Walter Lübeck

At practically every lecture that I hold on the topic of nutritional supplements, I am asked why something like this is necessary at all. Isn't it enough to think positively, eat whole foods, and engage in an exercise program on a regular basis? Over the years, I have given much thought to this topic. Today, this is my perspective on it:

During the last 200 years or so, a gigantic process of radical change has taken place for humanity. For the most part, this has occurred as a result of the Industrial Revolution. The environment has changed to an incredible extent within a very short period of time, seen in geological terms. Pesticides, insecticides, herbicides, fungicides, antibiotics, chemical fertilizers, preservatives and artificial dyes, solvents, fuels, and other poisons, as well as an intensely heightened level of environmental radioactivity and electrical and electromagnetic emanations from an immense number of constantly increasing sources, have a negative effect on the human body's metabolism—and many other things—to a degree entirely unknown before.

Humanity has changed—the stress has increased in an unnatural way.

Many of conventional medicine's medications that have been used on a wide-scale basis have frequently turned out to be remedies with very unpleasant effects in the long run. A further factor is a general shift to a lifestyle with increasingly higher demands on performance and more and more stress.

Our environmental situation has changed greatly as well. Instead of giant forests, meandering clean rivers, pure air, and a greatly diversified animal and plant world, today we have a landscape that is increasingly characterized by overdevelopment, asphalt, and canalization.

Conventional medicine's medications can have unpleasant side effects.

Despite all of these absolutely unaccustomed influences, the human body should also remain healthy and productive for several more decades so that life is worth living. If I look at things with this perspective, I find it totally illuminating that the metabolism needs a bit more than whole foods in order to be fit for the constantly demanded highest level of performance in our age. It is certainly absolutely appropriate to have a constructive

Athletes are enthusiastic about nutritional supplements—better and safer than anabolic drugs.

attitude toward life, keep our bodies fit with a healthy amount of sports, and eat a sensible diet. However, according to my experience and observations in my practice as a personal consultant and leader of seminars, all of this is no longer enough. Today, if you would like to remain vital and healthy for years to come, you need *additional* nutritional supplements in the form of vitamins and vitamin-like substances, minerals, trace elements, bioflavondoids, herbal extracts, fruit and vegetable extracts, and other good things of a similar nature. High-performance athletes all over the world are increasingly depending on this kind of help instead of anabolic drugs and other agents from the sorcerer's kitchen of chemistry, which may help in the short term but turn a healthy organism into a wreck in the long run.

Incidentally, this train of thought isn't new: Ultimately, the use of beef broth with its effective ingredient of L-carnitine as a traditional home remedy for a speedier recovery after the flu, the guarana that the Indians in South America have used for centuries as a healing remedy and energy-provider in times of great stress, the catuaba and pau d'arco that people have also enjoyed using since time immemorial in this part of the world, the tea-tree oil that Australia's Aborigines value greatly, the green tea that the Taoist and Buddhist monks like to drink, the Reishi mushroom in Japan—the list of these "classic" nutritional supplements could easily fill its own book. Basically, the only thing that is new is the thought of looking around the world to see what good things there are for improving health and performance and making them available to as many people as possible for the improvement of life quality without additional risks.

For centuries, people in all parts of the world have taken nutritional supplements to increase their quality of life.

People who reject nutritional supplements should give some thought to these facts. We can't turn back the hands of time. But we can—each of us for ourselves—take responsibility for surviving this increasingly complicated world in the best way possible. Only healthy people with great reserves have their full creative potential, their complete physical and psychological capacity available to them in order to find the paths out of our self-created ecological and social problems—and take them. A person who can no longer get on his or her feet because of illness and weakness also cannot walk through the nearby gates of paradise, even when they are open.

The challenges of life should be mastered with creativity and much joy.

I have personally decided not to suffer from problems but to master the challenges in my life as creatively and joyfully as possible.

What do you want to do with the years of life ahead of you: Suffer—or live?

Monograph: L-Carnitine
(from the German Federal Gazette No. 11
of January 17th, 1990)

Effective components: ASK.: 22107 L-Carnitine*
23634 L-Carnitine Hydrochloride

Pharmocological Properties,
Pharmacokinetics, Toxicology

L-carnitine is a quaternary amine compound physiologically occurring in the human organism. Its main function is transporting the activated long-chain fatty acids through the inner mitochondrial membrane into the mitochondria, where they are brought to the beta-oxidation process. In addition, it plays an important role in the ketogenisis of the liver. Substituting L-carnitine when there is an L-carnitine deficiency leads to an increased oxidation of fatty acids, resulting in an increase of ketogenesis, as well as an improved overall energy metabolism. This is also shown in an increase of muscle strength. Through the formation of L-carnitine esters, excess short-chain and branched-chain acyl groups can be transported out of the mitochondria into the cytosol. In the case of some congenital metabolic disorders, the elimination of pathological metabolites may be increased. There is a regeneration of coenzyme A (CoA) and energy metabolism is improved. After oral administration, the absorption of L-carnitine is greater than 90%.

The cytosol is the cell plasma and the place where glucose metabolism occurs in the cells. Metabolite is the name given to all substances occurring in cellular metabolism.

Clinical Data

1. Areas of Application
For substitution in cases of primary, systemic L-carnitine deficiency, as well as for secondary L-carnitine deficiency on the basis of congenital metabolic disorders. As a possible treatment for special forms of muscular dystrophy with lipid accumulation, which are based on a primary muscular L-carnitine deficiency.

2. Contraindications
No contraindications are currently known.

3. Side Effects
Side effects for L-carnitine are rare. When taken orally (especially in high doses), there were infrequent cases of nausea, vomiting, and diarrhea.

4. Special Precautions
None.

5. Use during Pregnancy and Lactation
There are no reports on experiences of use during pregnancy and breastfeeding. However, since this is an endogenous substance, no risks should be expected.

6. Medicinal and Other Interactions
There are no known interactions with other agents.

7. Dosage and Type of Application
Children should take between 25 and 100mg per kilogram of body weight orally or intravenously, divided into a number of doses. For adults, use up to 5 grams daily, orally or intravenously.

8. Overdose
No toxic effects are known for L-carnitine.

9. Special Warnings
None.

10. Effects on Drivers and Machine Operators
None.

Bibliography

Selected Titles on L-Carnitine

Crayhon R. (1998). *The Carnitine Miracle.* New York:M. Evans & Co.

Leibowitz, B.E. (1998). *L-Carnitine—The Energy Nutrient.* Good Health Guides. Keats: USA.

Hughes R.E. (University of Wales)(1993). *L-Carnitine—Some Nutritional and Historical Implications.* Edition Lonza.

R. Ferrari, S. Dimauro, G. Sherwood (1992). *L-Carnitine and Its Role in Medicine: From Function to Therapy.* London: Academic Press.

E. Kaiser & A. Lohninger (1987). *Carnitine—Its Role in Lung and Heart Disorders.* Basel Switzerland: Karger Verlag.

Selected Scientific Literature on L-Carnitine
My current book on L-carnitine has been conceptualized as an easily understandable, introductory work for those who are not specialists in the medical field. Nevertheless, I would like to give the reader with an interest in science the possibility of learning more about L-carnitine. So here is a list of literature on the topic requiring more advanced training in medicine.

There are currently more than 9,000 academic papers about L-carnitine. Every year, hundreds more are published since L-carnitine is a substance that arouses interest. Its spectrum of activity in relation to the promotion and stabilization of health is enormous and its tolerability is outstanding. Because of the amount of publications, I have only selected a few exemplary papers that I personally consider particularly informative or historically significant.

Borum, R. (1985). Role of Carnitine during Development. *Canadian Journal of Physiological Pharmacology,* vol. 63, pp. 571-576.

Borum, R., York, C. M., and Broquist, H. P. (1979). Carnitine Content of Liquid Formulas and Special Diets. *American Journal of Clinical Nutrition,* vol. 32, pp. 2272-2276.

Bremer, J. (1983). Carnitine—Metabolism and Functions. *Physiological Reviews,* vol. 63, pp. 1420-1480.

Broquist, P. and Borum P.R. (1982). Carnitine Biosynthesis, Nutritional Implications. *Advances in Nutritional Research,* vol. 4, pp. 181-204.

de Jong, J.W. & Ferrari, R. (1999). *The Carnitine System: A New Therapeutical Approach to Cardiovascular Diseases.* Deventer, The Netherlands: Kluwer Academic Publishers.

de Simone, C. & Famularo, G. (Editor) (1997). *Carnitine Today.* Texas: Landes Biosciences.

Fraenkel, G. and Friedman, S. (1957). Carnitine. *Vitamins and Hormones,* vol. 15, pp. 73-118. New York: Academic Press.

Fritz, I.B. (1963). Carnitine and Its Role in Fatty Acid Metabolism. *Advances in Lipid Research,* vol. 1, pp. 285-334.

Genger, H., Enzelsberger, H., and Salzer, H. (1988). L-Carnitine als Therapie der Plazentainsuffizienz–Erste Erfahrungen. *Geburtsh. u. Perinat.* 192, pp. 155-157.

Genger, H., Sevelda, P., Vytiska-binstorfer, H., Salzer, H., Legenstein, E., and Lohninger, A. (1988). L-Carnitin-Spiegel während der Schwangerschaft. *Geburtsh. u. Perinat.* 192, pp. 134-36.

Gulewitsch, W. and Krimberg, R. (1905). Zur Kenntnis der Extraktivstoffe der Muskel. Über das L-Carnitin. *Hoppe-Seylers Zeitschrift fuer physiologische Chemie,* vol. 45, pp. 326-330.

Hughes, R. E. (1988). Ascorbic Acid, Carnitine and Fatigue. *Medical Science Research,* vol. 15, pp. 721-723.

Hughes, R.E. (1982). The Vitamin C, Carnitine, Fatigue Relationship. *Vitamin C. Conference Proceedings.* Editors: Counsell, J.N. and Hornig, D.H. , pp. 75-86. London: Applied Science.

Khan, L. and Bamji, M.S. (1979). Tissue Carnitine Deficiency Due to Dietary Lysine Deficiency. *Journal of Nutrition,* vol. 109, pp. 24-31.

Lombard, K.A., Olson, A.L., Nelson, S.E. and Retouche, C.J.(1989). Carnitine Status of Lactoovovegetarians and Strict Vegetarian Adults and Children. *American Journal of Clinical Nutrition,* vol. 50, pp. 301-306.

Mitchell, M.E. (1978). Carnitine Metabolism in Human Subjects. I. Normal Metabolism. *The American Journal of Clincial Nutrition,* vol. 31, pp. 293-306.

Scholte, H.R. and de Jonge, P.C. (1987). Metabolism, Function and Transport of Carnitine in Health and Disease. *Carnitine in der Medizin,* pp. 21-59. Edited by R. Gitzelmann. Stuttgart: Schattauer Verlag.

Tao, R.C. and Yoshimura, N.N. (1980). Carnitine Metabolism and Its Application in Parenteral Nutrition. *Journal of Parenteral and Enteral Nutrition,* vol. 4, pp. 469-486.

Wolfram, G. (1982). Die Bedeutung von L-Carnitin in Fettstoffwechsel. *Fett in der parenteralen Ernaehrung: Symposium,* pp. 28-47. Editors: J. Eckart and G. Wolfram. Munich: Zuckschwert Verlag.

Additional Reading Recommendations:

Leutjohann, S. (1998). *The Healing Power of Black Cumin.* Twin Lakes, WI: Lotus Light/Shangri-La.

Sharamon S./Baginski B. (1991). *The Chakra Handbook.* Twin Lakes, WI: Lotus Light/Shangri-La.

Sharamon S. Baginski B. (1997). *The Healing Power of Grapefruit Seed.* Twin Lakes, WI: Lotus Light/Shangri-La.

Lübeck, W. (1994). *The Complete Reiki Handbook.* Twin Lakes, WI: Lotus Light/Shangri-La.

Lübeck, W. (1995). *Reiki for First Aid.* Twin Lakes, WI: Lotus Light/Shangri-La.

Lübeck, W. (1996). *Reiki—Way of the Heart.* Twin Lakes, WI: Lotus Light/Shangri-La.

Lübeck, W. (1997). *Rainbow Reiki.* Twin Lakes, WI: Lotus Light/Shangri-La.

Lübeck, W. (1998). *The Healing Power of Pau D'Arco.* Twin Lakes, WI: Lotus Light/Shangri-La.

Lübeck, W. (1998). *Pendulum Healing Handbook.* Twin Lakes, WI: Lotus Light/Shangri-La.

Lübeck, W. (2000). *Aura Healing Handbook,* Twin Lakes. WI: Lotus Press/Shangri-La.

Lübeck, W. (2000). *The Tao of Money.* Twin Lakes, WI: Lotus Press/Shangri-La.

Index

Further Titles Released by LOTUS PRESS • SHANGRI-LA

Barbara Simonsohn
Healing Power of Papaya
A Holistic Health Handbook on How to Avoid Acidosis, Allergies, and Health Disorders
In her lively and descriptive health handbook, best-selling German author Barbara Simonsohn shares knowledge that native peoples from all over the world have successfully practiced for centuries. The "power fruit" papaya is virtually a universal remedy with a large spectrum of anti-inflammatory effects against many health disorders and diseases.   224 pages · $15.95 · ISBN 0-914955-63-2

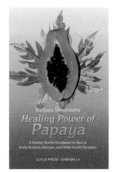

Thomas Dunkenberger
Tibetan Healing Handbook
A Practical Manual for Diagnosing, Treating, and Healing with Natural Tibetan Medicine
An introduction to one of the oldest healing systems: Tibetan natural medicine, comprehensive and easy to understand. The author informs you about the essential correlation and approaches taken by the Tibetan science of healing. It describes the entire spectrum of application possibilities for those who want to study Tibetan medicine and use it for treatment purposes.
240 pages · $15.95 · ISBN 0-914955-66-7

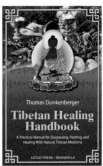

Andreas Jell
Healthy with Tachyon
A Complete Handbook Including Basic Principles and Application of Products for Health and Wellness
The comprehensive handbook for using tachyonized materials. A completely new chapter of human history has begun with the possibility of directly applying tachyon energy for healing and development. Today, you can directly strengthen your powers of self-healing by using tachyonized materials. These powers will then organize perfect healing and development (anti-entropy) through their own dynamic.   144 pages · $12.95 · ISBN 0-914955-58-6

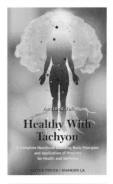

Wilhelm Gerstung · Jens Melhase
The Complete Feng Shui Health Handbook
How You Can Protect Yourself Against Harmful Energies and Create Positive Forces for Health and Prosperity
This fascinating handbook provides a wealth of graphics and practical information, which help design every home in such a way that it becomes a source of energy, allowing everybody to relax and re-energize himself. The authors integrate their many years of research and extensive knowledge of energies in the home, and particularly the sleeping area, with the Western science of underground watercourses and grids.   224 pages · $16.95 · ISBN 0914955-60-8

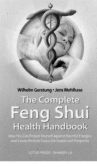

Further Titles Released by LOTUS PRESS • SHANGRI-LA

Dr. Mikao Usui and Frank Arjava Petter
The Original Reiki Handbook of Dr. Mikao Usui
The Traditional Usui Reiki Ryoho Treatment Positions and Numerous Reiki Techniques for Health and Well-Being
For the first time available outside of Japan. The original hand positions and healing techniques from Dr. Usui's handbook have been listed in detail, making it a valuable reference work for anyone who practices Reiki. Whether you are an initiate or a master, if you practice Reiki you can expand your knowledge dramatically as you follow in the footsteps of a great healer.

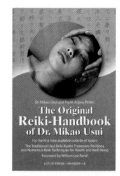

80 pages ·100 photos · $14.95 · ISBN 0-914955-57-8

Sylvia Luetjohann
The Healing Power of Black Cumin
A Handbook on Oriental Black Cumin Oils, Their Healing Components, and Special Recipes
Long confirmed by good experiences, the sensational effects of black oils have also been substantiated by modern science. Black cumin is an excellent healer. Its areas of application extend from skin care to the treatment of diseases of the skin and respiratory tract. The author describes the most important types of black cumin oils with their specific effects through the use of many practical examples.

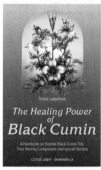

(Lotus Light) 160 pages · $14.95 · ISBN 0-914955-53-5

Walter Lübeck
The Healing Power of Pau D'Arco
The Divine Tree of the South American Shamans Provides Extraordinary Healing Benefits
This traditional naturopathic remedy of the Indios, is one of the most effective, economical, versatile, and pleasant-tasting remedies against a variety of acute and chronic health disorders. The components of the lapacho (pau d'arco) bark have a detoxifying, antimycotic, and anticarcinogenic effect, as well as being suitable for many chronic problems in particular. In addition, the bark has no side effects and is quite tasty. Walter Lübeck presents the best recipes for using the tea effectively.

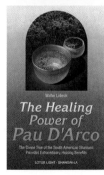

(Lotus Light) 132 pages · $12.95 · ISBN 0-914955-52-7

Shalila Sharamon · Bodo J. Baginski
The Healing Power of Grapefruit Seed
The Practical Handbook for Using Grapefruit Seed Extract to Heal Infections, Allergies, and Much More. One of the Most Effective New Healing Remedies
Based on international research, two bestselling authors have compiled sensational therapy successes and areas of application for this biological broad-spectrum therapeutic agent, antibiotic, antimycotic and antiparasitic, preservative, and hygienic agent of the future. In addition to scientific proof, this practice-oriented book includes proper dosages and procedures.

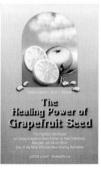

(Lotus Light) 160 pages · $12.95 · ISBN 0-914955-27-6

Herbs and other natural health products and information are often available at natural food stores or metaphysical bookstores. If you cannot find what you need locally, you can contact one of the following sources of supply.

Sources of Supply:

The following companies have an extensive selection of useful products and a long track-record of fulfillment. They have natural body care, aromatherapy, flower essences, crystals and tumbled stones, homeopathy, herbal products, vitamins and supplements, videos, books, audio tapes, candles, incense and bulk herbs, teas, massage tools and products and numerous alternative health items across a wide range of categories.

WHOLESALE:

Wholesale suppliers sell to stores and practitioners, not to individual consumers buying for their own personal use. Individual consumers should contact the RETAIL supplier listed below. Wholesale accounts should contact with business name, resale number or practitioner license in order to obtain a wholesale catalog and set up an account.

Lotus Light Enterprises, Inc.

P. O. Box 1008
Silver Lake, WI 531 70 USA
262 889 8501 (phone)
262 889 8591 (fax)
800 548 3824 (toll free order line)

RETAIL:

Retail suppliers provide products by mail order direct to consumers for their personal use. Stores or practitioners should contact the wholesale supplier listed above.

Internatural

33719 116th Street
Twin Lakes, WI 53181 USA
800 643 4221 (toll free order line)
262 889 8581 office phone
WEB SITE: www.internatural.com

Web site includes an extensive annotated catalog of more than 7000 products that can be ordered "on line" for your convenience 24 hours a day, 7 days a week.